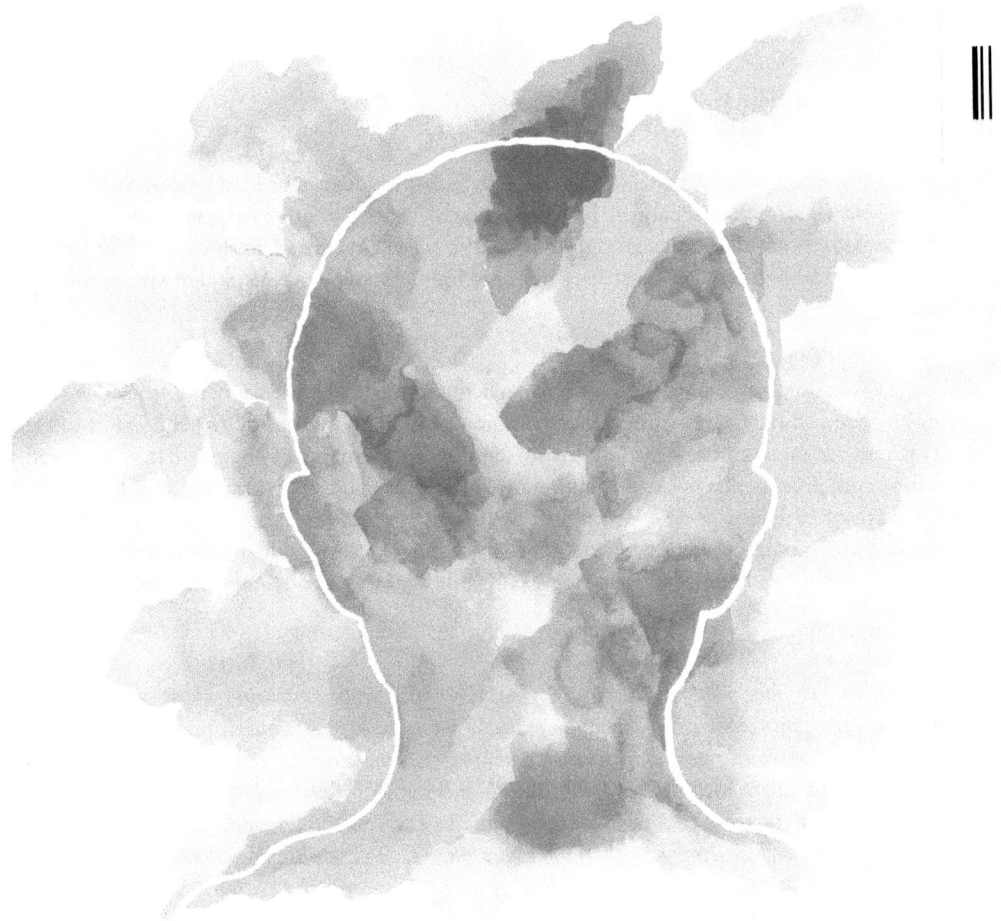

The Influence of Psychological Trauma
in Nursing

INSTRUCTOR'S GUIDE

Karen J. Foli, PhD, RN, FAAN

John R. Thompson, MD

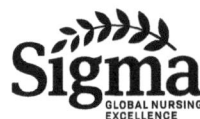

The Sigma Theta Tau International Honor Society of Nursing (Sigma) is a nonprofit organization whose mission is advancing world health and celebrating nursing excellence in scholarship, leadership, and service. Founded in 1922, Sigma has more than 135,000 active members in over 90 countries and territories. Members include practicing nurses, instructors, researchers, policymakers, entrepreneurs, and others. Sigma's more than 530 chapters are located at more than 700 institutions of higher education throughout Armenia, Australia, Botswana, Brazil, Canada, Colombia, England, Ghana, Hong Kong, Ireland, Japan, Jordan, Kenya, Lebanon, Malawi, Mexico, the Netherlands, Nigeria, Pakistan, Philippines, Portugal, Puerto Rico, Singapore, South Africa, South Korea, Swaziland, Sweden, Taiwan, Tanzania, Thailand, the United States, and Wales. Learn more at www.sigmanursing.org.

Sigma Theta Tau International
550 West North Street
Indianapolis, IN, USA 46202

To order additional books, buy in bulk, or order for corporate use, contact Sigma Marketplace at 888.654.4968 (US and Canada) or +1.317.634.8171 (outside US and Canada).

To request a review copy for course adoption, email solutions@sigmamarketplace.org or call 888.654.4968 (US and Canada) or +1.317.634.8171 (outside US and Canada).

To request author information, or for speaker or other media requests, contact Sigma Marketing at 888.634.7575 (US and Canada) or +1.317.634.8171 (outside US and Canada).

Print ISBN: 9781948057059
PDF ISBN: 9781948057042

Publisher: Dustin Sullivan
Acquisitions Editor: Emily Hatch
Cover Designer: Rebecca Batchelor
Interior Design/Page Layout: Rebecca Batchelor

Managing Editor: Carla Hall
Development and Project Editor: Rebecca Senninger
Copy Editor: Gill Editorial Services
Proofreader: Todd Lothery

DEDICATION

This instructor's guide is dedicated to nurses who seek healing
from trauma within themselves and who
seek healing for others.

ACKNOWLEDGMENTS

The goal of any work is to ensure that the aim and audience are always kept in the center of the authors' efforts. Our aim—to increase insight into personal trauma and build trauma awareness and resilience in new nurses—was always in the forefront of our energies. As we sought to secure a home for this book, we believed this book was needed and would ultimately improve the quality of nurses' lives and enhance patient-centered care.

We are grateful to Sigma and its publishing staff. To Emily Hatch, thank you for our first meeting during which you advised Karen to think more broadly in nursing education, while focusing the work. To Carla Hall, for encouragement, great communication throughout the process, and assisting with book graphics and permissions. To Dustin Sullivan, who supported and celebrated with us as we completed this book. And finally, to the Sigma publishing committee, who requested companion books so that students could apply trauma-informed nursing care through simulations. In summary, thank you for believing in this book.

Specific to the instructor's guide and student workbook, we extend a special acknowledgment to the National League for Nursing for allowing us to adapt its Simulation Design Template, which was originally adapted from the work of Childs, Sepples, and Chambers (2007). We greatly appreciate their generosity in allowing us to use this intellectual property.

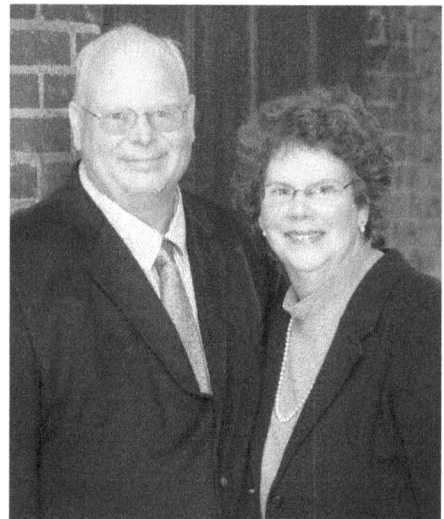

ABOUT THE AUTHORS

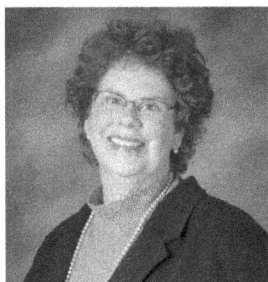

Karen J. Foli, PhD, RN, FAAN, received her associate's and bachelor's degrees from Indiana State University and her master's degree, with an emphasis in nursing administration, from Indiana University School of Nursing, Indianapolis. Dr. Foli received her PhD in communications from the University of Illinois, Urbana–Champaign. She is an Associate Professor and the Director of the PhD in Nursing Program at Purdue University School of Nursing, West Lafayette, Indiana.

Foli is a fellow in the American Academy of Nursing (AAN) in recognition for her work with nontraditional families, such as adoption and kinship families. She is a member of the Child, Adolescent, and Family Expert Panel through the AAN. She has forwarded a mid-range theory of parental postadoption depression and has tested this theory in empirical studies. Her research is bound together to alleviate the suffering of psychological trauma. She is currently examining the role of psychological trauma in substance use in registered nurses.

A recipient of numerous teaching awards, including the Charles B. Murphy Outstanding Undergraduate Teaching Award from Purdue University, the highest award bestowed for undergraduate teaching at the university, Foli takes pride in being a nurse educator. In 2018, she was one of 45 faculty members who were inducted into the Purdue University Book of Great Teachers, signifying excellence in teaching. She also received the Sigma Theta Tau International Honor Society of Nursing Delta Omicron Chapter Award for Outstanding Mentoring in 2017. Preparing nurse scientists is also an important part of Foli's professional work. As the director of the PhD in Nursing Program, she encourages and guides students and faculty in preparing nurses who will continue to explore and build upon the science of nursing.

Foli's lifelong love of writing has produced works in a wide range of formats and genres, including memoir, regulatory writing in the pharmaceutical industry, scholarly writing of empirical studies, and mystery short stories. She is author or coauthor of four well-received health-related books. One of these, *Nursing Care of Adoption and Kinship Families: A Clinical Guide for Advanced Practice Nurses* (2017, Springer), received the American Psychiatric Nurses Association (APNA) Award for Media in 2018. This award "recognizes APNA members who have demonstrated excellence in producing media related to psychiatric-mental health nursing."

A special passion of Foli's work is advancing the conceptualization of nursing and the "work" of nurses. The elusive definition of nursing motivates her efforts to forward a way to value and communicate what nurses do in practice, in education, in policy, and in research. She has partnered with many graduate students and coauthored several papers that define important concepts surrounding nursing care.

Her appreciation for nurses and the profession of nursing is unique in that her career path veered away from the profession for a time and carried her into professional writing, teaching business communications in a Big Ten business school, and writing global experimental research protocols for a large pharmaceutical company. When she returned to the world of nursing, Foli realized how much society needs the special comfort, caring, and compassion offered by nurses. Her deep appreciation for what nurses experience motivated her to write this book to prepare students and those new to the field to become stronger and more resilient as they process and encounter patients in crises and in need of trauma-informed care.

———————

Foli and her coauthor, John R. Thompson, have been married for almost three decades and have three adult children. Avid dog lovers, they have always been owners of at least three dogs, many times taking in strays and "dumped" animals who became loved members of their family.

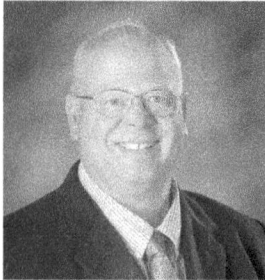

John R. Thompson, MD, has practiced as a physician in the specialty area of psychiatry for the past 30 years. He completed his residency in general psychiatry and a fellowship in child/adolescent psychiatry in the Department of Psychiatry at Indiana University. Since Thompson's fellowship, he has worked with a variety of populations, including children, adolescents, young adults, and adults, including addiction psychiatry. He has practiced in multiple healthcare contexts: acute care/inpatient care, intensive outpatient, community mental health, consult-liaison, veterans' mental health, and forensic psychiatry. Along with Karen Foli, he is coauthor of *The Post-Adoption Blues: Overcoming the Unforeseen Challenges of Adoption* (Rodale, 2004).

Currently, he practices psychiatric medicine for Purdue University's Counseling and Psychological Services, West Lafayette, Indiana. In this position, Thompson evaluates and manages the psychiatric needs of students enrolled in higher education. Common issues include depression, anxiety, substance use, personality disorders, attention deficit disorder, and healing from trauma.

Thompson is also a cancer survivor; thus, his insights into trauma are both personal and professional. In his medical practice, he assesses and counsels young adults who are processing and recovering from trauma. Thompson approaches the individual in a trauma-informed, holistic way. He strives to promote a feeling of safety and allows the individual to share past experiences as the relationship is built and trust evolves. He believes in "de-prescribing" medications—removing those agents that create addictions, lack a therapeutic rationale, or are interacting with other agents in nontherapeutic ways. Taking time to review medical records, Thompson pieces together past traumas, dual diagnoses, and concurrent medical conditions that, when revealed, contribute to optimal care. Recognizing that healthcare disparities and social determinants of health result in individuals struggling to secure resources in filling prescriptions and in the wider community, he searches for affordable healthcare and orders appropriate referrals to provide for a continuum of care.

Growing up in the Rocky Mountains of Colorado, Thompson enjoys nature and being outdoors. His spirit is recharged upon seeing growth both in his plants and trees, and more importantly, in people. Being part of students' success, seeing them achieve their career goals as they develop as young adults, motivates Thompson to continue to offer each individual his best efforts as a medical provider.

THE INFLUENCE OF PSYCHOLOGICAL TRAUMA IN NURSING

INSTRUCTOR'S GUIDE

TABLE OF CONTENTS

INTRODUCTION

In nursing as well as in healthcare, the topic of "trauma-informed care" is discussed frequently. This type of approach is characterized by the caregiver being knowledgeable about psychological trauma and strategies to mitigate its effects. For the instructor, being aware of all of your students' pasts is typically not possible; it is also not desirable. It is important, however, when we begin to discuss simulations surrounding psychological trauma that we understand the role of faculty. Clarity of faculty roles is significant. Although at times you may feel as if you are a therapist to your students, that isn't your primary role. However, your students may react to the simulations in ways that are unexpected and unpredictable.

When Karen was a clinical instructor for a psychiatric mental health nursing course, students would often experience traumatic triggers or observe events that disturbed or frightened them. Several of Karen's students were adult learners, with the school located in a rural Illinois community. One student in particular stood apart from the rest. Diane was in her early thirties, married with two small children. Her face reflected a hard life, and this education meant a better existence for her and her children. At the beginning of the semester, Diane's appearance was characterized by short, straight, brown hair; extra weight; and casual dress. As the weeks progressed and Diane began to interact with inpatients on the psychiatric unit, including women who had experienced domestic violence, her appearance began to change. She lost weight and frosted and curled her hair. Her affect changed as well, with more smiles and animated speech. Finally, Karen commented on the changes. She turned to Karen and said:

"I finally left him. I realized I didn't have to take it anymore. Speaking to those patients, I thought, 'I better take my own advice.'"

Diane then described an abusive relationship she'd endured for years with her husband. The nursing care she had been absorbing and internalizing had spilled into her personal world, and she found the motivation and resources to finally change her situation. This is only one example of how students are affected by what they learn in class, clinical, and from the peers and patients they interact with. This extraordinarily resilient woman chose a different path once she became aware of how psychological trauma affected individuals and her own life.

PURPOSE AND STRUCTURE

This instructor's guide is designed as a companion to the primary book, *The Influence of Psychological Trauma in Nursing,* which digs deep into psychological trauma in nursing and approaches to healing. The purpose of the instructor's guide is to provide content for the nurse educator surrounding best educational practices to support students who have experienced psychological trauma and to ready students for the trauma they will experience as professional nurses. The simulations are based on composite cases; therefore, they do not represent any specific individual. Still, students may be inclined to identify themselves or someone they know in these scenarios. Also, the guide serves to present simulation activities that may be used as stand-alone activities or complementary simulations with other materials you may already be using. Our hope is that this guide will not only prepare nurses and support compassionate care and resiliency, but also inform you as a person, an educator, and a nurse about the often-overlooked influences of psychological trauma in your professional life.

PEDAGOGICAL CONSIDERATIONS IN SIMULATIONS SURROUNDING PSYCHOLOGICAL TRAUMA

During the beginning of these simulation activities, students will need to be grounded in a new vocabulary about psychological trauma, and, depending upon which course this guide will be used for, simulation may also be new to the student. Although simulation has become an accepted proxy for student clinical experiences, often empirical knowledge of the sciences is discussed first and foremost. Laboratory values, physical assessments, medication mechanisms of actions/interactions, and prompts to seek other healthcare providers characterize many simulation activities. The following simulations, in contrast and to a great extent, focus upon the psychological, social, emotional, and spiritual dimensions during and after trauma.

When implementing simulations about trauma-informed care, the instructor will need to "practice what is preached": The environment has to be perceived as safe, comfortably controlled, and supportive of peer-to-peer and student-to-faculty connections. The next responsibility will be to have the students grasp and apply interventions that are informed by reactions to trauma. We start with a discussion of trauma-informed care, and then we move to issues surrounding simulations focused on trauma and trauma-informed interventions.

PSYCHOLOGICAL TRAUMA

Depending upon the population of students you serve, maturity and development affect how they see trauma. For example, as adolescent and young adult brains' prefrontal cortexes mature, there is less impulsivity and the ability to be increasingly mindful. Therefore, trauma needs to be well defined and conceptualized to be meaningful. What trauma is not may be as important a group discussion as what trauma is. The Substance Abuse and Mental Health Services Administration (SAMHSA, 2014a, n.p.) refers to trauma as:

> experiences that cause intense physical and psychological stress reactions. It can refer to a
> single event, multiple events, or a set of circumstances that is experienced by an individual
> as physically and emotionally harmful or threatening and that has lasting adverse effects on
> the individual's physical, social, emotional, or spiritual well-being.

According to this definition, an intense stress reaction is experienced based on one or several events. Such experiences potentially create lasting effects on the individual. There are times when trauma is not linked to the threat of physical harm; it is intensely perceived harm from a psychological perspective. The individual nature of how we react to and process trauma is also of note. Several buffers that mitigate trauma exist, including one's resiliency.

In Figure 1.1, we conceptualize trauma from both individual and nurse-specific perspectives. In this instructor's guide, the six simulations concentrate on those events most likely to be encountered by student nurses and those new to the profession. Three sections divide the guide temporally and by role: the student nurse during college (student and peers), the student during college (student as new caregiver), and after graduation (new nurse in the workforce). Specifically, the six simulations address the trauma of bullying (centered around sexual minority status), posttraumatic stress disorder (PTSD; veteran experiencing post-traumatic stress symptoms), second-victim trauma (student nurse who makes a medication error), secondary traumatic stress (student nurse witnesses unexpected death), system-induced trauma (patient who is agitated and nonadherent), and workplace violence (new nurse who has been injured by patient). Many of these types of trauma can be located on the right side of the trauma circle in Figure 1.1.

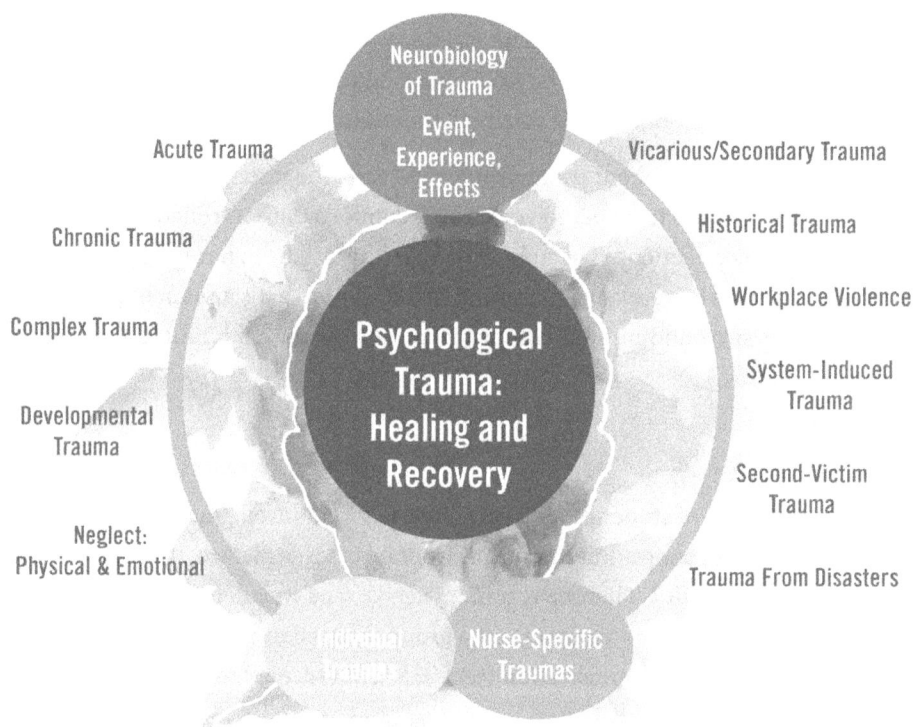

FIGURE 1.1 Conceptualizing trauma.

We metaphorically toss the term "trauma-informed" around in our vocabulary, but what does this mean for caregivers? We found a definition that is comprehensive and incorporates the goals of being trauma-informed:

> (1) to understand how violence and victimization have figured in the lives of most consumers of mental health, substance abuse, and other services and (2) to apply that understanding in providing services and designing service systems so that they accommodate the needs and vulnerabilities of trauma survivors and facilitate client participation in treatment. (Butler, Critelli, & Rinfrette, 2011, p. 178)

We appreciate this definition of trauma-informed care and would modify it slightly to include caregivers/ nurses who may experience trauma. The systems nurses work in also need to be designed to prevent and mitigate the experiences of traumatic events for both patients and nurses.

When an individual has experienced trauma, the Event, Experience, and Effects (SAMHSA, 2014b) are filtered on an individual level. How these three areas are processed depends on multiple factors, including a history of trauma, support systems, and personal buffers such as resiliency. In this way, students will also live through and process trauma in unique ways. As faculty, you need to be aware of the individualized signs and symptoms of posttraumatic stress, which these simulations may evoke in your students.

SIMULATION

To be clear, this is not a guide about how to design, implement, and evaluate simulation activities. That being said, this instructor's guide addresses aspects of simulation scenarios that take a unique approach due to the subject of trauma. For example, the issue of standardized patients (SPs) and securing those individuals is distinct with these simulations. For further discussion on simulations, we refer the reader to organizations such as the International Nursing Association for Clinical Simulation and Learning (INACSL), the Society for Simulation in Healthcare, and the Association of Standardized Patient Educators (ASPE). The National Councils of State Boards of Nursing also discuss the use of simulation in prelicensure programs. Specific contributions from the internationally renowned Pamela R. Jeffries, PhD, RN, FAAN, ANEF, who has forwarded evidence, as well as theory on simulation in nursing, are noteworthy.

One important reminder is that all simulations need to be integrated into the curriculum and linked back to course and program objectives. Our major thesis is that psychological trauma is a thread throughout the interface between peers, patients, and faculty in nursing curricula. These materials are written at the level of beginning nursing students, but they are certainly adaptable to more experienced students.

RULE #1: PSYCHOLOGICAL SAFETY

Faculty need to be aware of how to make students feel safe before, during, and after simulation. As we've discussed, simulation exercises may trigger past traumas and emotions. In a concept analysis of psychological safety during high-fidelity simulation, Turner and Harder (2018) define this concept as:

> A feeling or climate whereby the learner can feel valued and comfortable yet still speak up
> and take risks without fear of retribution, embarrassment, judgment or consequences either
> to themselves or others, thereby promoting learning and innovation. (p. 49)

Three defining attributes are offered: The student has the ability to make errors without consequences; the facilitator has qualities that promote and preserve a safe environment; and prelearning activities, such as orientation, preparation, objectives, and expectations, are clear (Turner & Harder, 2018, p. 47). When conducting simulations with a trauma focus and frequently SPs, there are additional considerations, such as trauma triggers and the aftereffects of the simulation, that may create intrusive thoughts related to the trauma. In addition, faculty need to be sensitive to retraumatization as a result of the simulation. Therefore, to ensure the provision of a psychologically safe environment prior to, during, and post simulations that present trauma-related materials, faculty should:

1. Be knowledgeable about available internal and external resources for the student should the student need psychological support as a result of the prework, real-time simulation, and post-simulation (school counselors/advisors, counseling services in the larger organization, and so forth).

2. Emphasize to the student group that content may be sensitive to some of their peers and this is an opportunity to provide trauma-informed care within the student group.

3. Review salient concepts such as feelings of safety, compassion, resiliency, posttraumatic growth, and healing as part of the simulations.

4. Allow students to exit the simulation and continue debriefing at their own pace without consequences if there is psychological distress.

5. Firmly reiterate the confidentiality of the group discussion; however, faculty should also clarify that personal sharing is not mandatory and should be done within the context of the simulation scenario.

6. Understand that individual and group debriefing may occur after the formal discussion ends. As appropriate, be available to students who need to continue to process the experience.

SIMULATION PREPARATION

In alignment with nursing educational principles, preparation is paramount to pedagogical effectiveness. Due to the sensitive nature of trauma-related simulations, such preparation not only supports educational best practices, but also mitigates the risk of exposing students to further trauma. Next, we've highlighted several important factors to consider when implementing the simulations outlined in this instructor's guide.

STANDARDIZED PATIENTS AND SAFETY RULES

From a fidelity standpoint, the simulations that are psychiatric in nature or focused on mental health usually do not involve manikins. Either live actors or SPs are typically used to depict the learning situation. Anecdotally, some schools may use course faculty to act in psychiatric simulations. Many would argue against this practice based upon the dual responsibility of portraying the psychological impact of the scenario and being able to evaluate student performance. Also, students may have difficulty in believing that the faculty member is truly experiencing mental distress, thus impacting fidelity.

Options to secure SPs include training and engaging:

- Nursing faculty (who will not be evaluating students and are therefore divorced from the class) or volunteers from centers for teaching and learning

- Undergraduate or graduate nursing students who are not involved in the course

---

- Students in other departments at your educational organization, including theater students
- Paid, live actors

The preparation of these individuals is critical to the simulations' success and, as importantly, the safety that the student perceives. ASPE has established standards of best practices, which are to be used in conjunction with the INACSL simulations standards. Standardized or simulated participants are to provide consistent and accurate portrayals of the patients within the learning contexts provided. Lewis et al. (2017) forwarded five domains of best practices when using standardized/simulated patients:

1. **Safe work environment:** Assurance of safety to all individuals involved in the simulation; quality, professionalism, and accountability

2. **Case development:** Preparation of the simulation with learning objectives in mind and using guidance from simulation organizations for case components

3. **SP training:** Role portrayal, feedback, and completion of assessment instruments

4. **Program management:** Purpose statement of the program, and clear policies and procedures

5. **Professional development:** Career development and leadership

In terms of simulations related to trauma, the first domain—safety—is of utmost importance. Ensuring confidentiality of the simulation experience, adequate training, reporting of conflicts of interest, and outlining when termination of the activity could occur if deemed unsafe are all necessary (Lewis et al., 2017). Similarly, the training of SPs must take into account past trauma that may affect their role in simulation, including their trauma triggers. Educators should address whether feedback, if offered by SPs, is offered without bias, which may be influenced by the students' roles in the scenario. Taken as a whole, simulations with SPs should be seen as a program with policies and procedures to guide educators, as well as plans for ongoing professional development (Lewis et al., 2017).

PREBRIEFING

For each of the six simulations in this instructor's guide, a foundation of understanding the nature of the activity (trauma-focused) should be communicated prior to the event. Transparency and clarity of the learning objectives (usually about two or three) are needed for the faculty and students to measure the impact of the simulation exercise. At times, part of the learning is for the students to discern the trauma context. Frequently, they will gravitate toward the empirical and task-oriented materials. Faculty will want to review *The Influence of Psychological Trauma in Nursing: Student Workbook* to decide whether the preparation materials are sufficient to design an optimal learning environment. We sought to provide enough information to allow the students to prepare for the simulation without sacrificing their ability to engage in spontaneous learning as the activity unfolds. (Note: The student workbook prebriefing content is abbreviated from what is included in this faculty guide.)

In addition to prebriefing information, for each trauma-focused simulation, students need to review:

- Basic therapeutic communications skills

- The definitions of trauma (see SAMHSA, 2014a) and trauma-informed care (Butler et al., 2011)

- The types of trauma specific to nursing (see Figure 1.1)

- The scenario from a micro (individual) and macro (system) perspective

- The six guiding principles of trauma-informed care (see Table 1.1)

These guiding principles (SAMHSA, 2014b) encapsulate much of what we've previously described. Safety is paramount for students, SPs, and faculty. The risks of retraumatization should be strategically minimized as the lesson unfolds. Faculty and peers should be viewed as trustworthy; students should appreciate that faculty have guided their learning in a spirit of transparency and candidness. Peer support and mutual self-help serve as opportunities to practice skills, such as therapeutic communication techniques within a trauma-informed framework. For example, our language creates reality and our questions do as well. It is important to ask those who have experienced or witnessed trauma, "What has happened to you?" versus "What is wrong with you?" (SAMHSA-HRSA Center for Integrated Health Solutions, n.d.).

TABLE 1.1   SAMHSA'S SIX GUIDING PRINCIPLES OF TRAUMA-INFORMED CARE

Principle 1: Safety
Principle 2: Trustworthiness and transparency
Principle 3: Peer support and mutual self-help
Principle 4: Collaboration and mutuality
Principle 5: Empowerment, voice, and choice
Principle 6: Cultural, historical, and gender issues

Source: SAMHSA, 2014b

Student and early career nurses should be socialized to the norm of collaboration and support for peers and patients. In this way, individuals will feel more empowered, own their voices, realize there are choices to move toward healing and recovery, and build resilience. Cultural, historical, and gender factors affect how trauma is interpreted with certain groups vulnerable to trauma in different circumstances and settings. Understanding social determinants of health, examining nursing theories, and valuing historical/intergenerational trauma will influence how effectively we appreciate these distinctions.

DURING

Scripts are provided in the simulations in this instructor's guide. Although a complete verbatim dialogue isn't desired or feasible, the script provides a beginning and ending to the activity. The language sets the tone for the scenarios. We've outlined the roles in the preceding text: SPs, students as both observers and participants, and faculty as facilitators and guides. With simulations surrounding lessons about trauma-informed care, faculty must be vigilant about cues to student distress. Competent faculty assessments, and reactions to students' affect and its relationship to learning, will be key to individuals' safety. Allowing students to disengage without penalty is an example of how to provide comfort.

DEBRIEFING

Faculty involved in simulation learning have often commented how powerful debriefing can be—some would argue this is when the significant value of simulations emerges. In this context, the goals of debriefing are to have 1) students learn the knowledge, apply the skills, and socialize to the attitudes inherent in trauma-informed care toward patients, peers, and self; and 2) faculty practice trauma-informed care toward students as trauma histories surface. There are several models to effective debriefing, and most likely, you have one that is preferred. We encourage you to take this model and conceptually map it to the principles of trauma-informed care. With permission, we've used the Simulation Design Template (National League for Nursing, 2018) to structure the learning activities. This template includes each component of a simulation; however, select parts have been deleted if they did not apply to the situation. After each simulation, we've included a link to the original template for your review. Last, we encourage you to be attuned to your own trauma scripts; you may be surprised as your own feelings surface based on what has happened to you in life.

ADDITIONAL THOUGHTS

The six simulations are structured as the student nurse moves forward in his or her career and changes roles, from student to newly licensed professional. The following simulations may be stand-alone activities or components to other simulations. For example, in the case of the student witnessing his first patient death, a paired simulation may be about the cause of death (postpartum hemorrhage). Similarly, the simulation focused on second-victim trauma (medication error) could be integrated with a lab on medication administration. In terms of course placement, we would caution against shifting these simulations to only psychiatric nursing courses. Practicing nurses clearly appreciate how behavioral health issues are infused in all areas of patient care delivery. Thus, we want students and newly practicing nurses to internalize the value of compassionate care to those peers and patients who are experiencing traumatic events or who have residual stress from past trauma.

REFERENCES

Butler, L. D., Critelli, F. M., & Rinfrette, E. S. (2011). Trauma-informed care and mental health. *Directions in Psychiatry, 31*, 197–210.

Lewis, K. L., Bohnert, C. A., Gammon, W. L., Hölzer, H., Lyman, L., Smith, C., . . . Gliva-McConvey, G. (2017). The Association of Standardized Patient Educators (ASPE) standards of best practice (SOBP). *Advances in Simulation, 2*(10). doi: https://doi.org/10.1186/s41077-017-0043-4

National League for Nursing. (2018). Simulation Design Template. Washington, DC: Author. Retrieved from https://sirc.nln.org/pluginfile.php/18733/mod_page/content/51/Simulation%20Design%20Template%202018.docx

SAMHSA-HRSA Center for Integrated Health Solutions. (n.d.). Trauma. Retrieved from https://www.integration.samhsa.gov/clinical-practice/trauma-informed

Substance Abuse and Mental Health Services Administration. (2014a). Key terms: Definitions. *SAMHSA News, 22*(2). Retrieved from https://www.samhsa.gov/samhsaNewsLetter/Volume_22_Number_2/trauma_tip/key_terms.html

Substance Abuse and Mental Health Services Administration. (2014b). *SAMHSA's concept of trauma and guidance for a trauma-informed approach.* HHS Publication No. (SMA) 14-4884. Rockville, MD: Author.

Turner, S., & Harder, N. (2018). Psychological safe environment: A concept analysis. *Clinical Simulation in Nursing, 18*, 47–55. doi: https://doi.org/10.1016/j.ecns.2018.02.004

SECTION 1

TRAUMA DURING COLLEGE:
THE STUDENT NURSE AND PEERS

INTERPERSONAL TRAUMA: SEXUAL IDENTITY BULLYING

A transgender individual (male-to-female; MTF), Khris is in her sophomore year of nursing and has been assigned an observation day in the operating room with other student nurses. While changing, two peers observe that Khris still has the anatomy of a biological male. Unknown to her peers, Khris has a history of harassment and bullying from peers, and she attempted suicide (ingestion of mother's benzodiazepine) during her freshman year of high school.

This simulation concentrates on an individual's sexual identity being exposed in a traumatic way. The clinical group of peers is the social unit under examination in this exercise. The goal is to translate trauma-informed knowledge, skills, and attitudes to sexual minority patients whom the students and new nurses will encounter as caregivers.

SIMULATION 1

DISCIPLINE: Nursing

EXPECTED SIMULATION RUN TIME:
15–20 minutes

LOCATION: Simulation lab

TODAY'S DATE: _____

FILE NAME: Khris

STUDENT LEVEL: Undergraduate nursing student

GUIDED REFLECTION TIME: Twice the amount of time that the simulation runs

LOCATION FOR REFLECTION: Simulation lab quiet room

BRIEF DESCRIPTION OF INDIVIDUAL

NAME: Khris Smith

DATE OF BIRTH: 03/22/2000

GENDER: Trans (MTF) **AGE:** 20 years **WEIGHT:** 150 pounds **HEIGHT:** 5'7"

RACE: White **RELIGION:** Agnostic

MAJOR SUPPORT: LGBTQ Community Center on campus

PAST MEDICAL HISTORY: Sophomore; decided to undergo hormonal therapy to transition from a male to a female. She has been receiving medical treatments to complete this gender transformation for the past 18 months.

HISTORY OF PRESENT ILLNESS: N/A

SOCIAL HISTORY: Khris was isolated from peers during high school. Has a past history of suicide attempt x 1 during freshman year of high school.

PRIMARY MEDICAL DIAGNOSIS: N/A

SURGERIES/PROCEDURES & DATES: Under physician care for transitioning, MTF, with hormonal therapy

PSYCHOMOTOR SKILLS REQUIRED OF PARTICIPANTS PRIOR TO SIMULATION

None

COGNITIVE ACTIVITIES REQUIRED OF PARTICIPANTS PRIOR TO SIMULATION

PRIOR TO THE SIMULATION, THE STUDENT SHOULD:

WATCH THE VIDEOS:

- GLSEN. (2017). *How to support transgender students.* Retrieved from https://www.youtube.com/watch?v=kq19QdOfH1Y

- The National Child Traumatic Stress Network. (2015). *Safe places, safe spaces: Creating welcoming and inclusive environments for traumatized LGBTQ youth.* Retrieved from https://www.nctsn.org/resources/safe-places-safe-spaces-creating-welcoming-and-inclusive-environments-traumatized-lgbtq-0

READ:

Aul, K. (2017). Who's uncivil to who? Perceptions of incivility in pre-licensure nursing programs. *Nursing Education in Practice, 27,* 36–44. doi: http://dx.doi.org/10.1016/j.nepr.2017.08.016

El-Azeem Ibrahim, S. A., & Ahmed Qalawa, S. (2016). Factors affecting nursing students' incivility: As perceived by students and faculty staff. *Nurse Education Today, 36,* 118–123. doi: http://dx.doi.org/10.1016/j.nedt.2015.08.014

National Child Traumatic Stress Network, Child Sexual Abuse Collaborative Group. (2014). *LGBTQ youth and sexual abuse: Information for mental health professionals.* Los Angeles, CA, and Durham, NC: National Center for Child Traumatic Stress. Retrieved from https://www.nctsn.org/sites/default/files/resources//lgbtq_youth_sexual_abuse_professionals.pdf

SIMULATION LEARNING OBJECTIVES

1. Employ strategies to reduce risk of harm to peers.

2. Communicate with peers in a manner that illustrates caring, reflects cultural awareness, and addresses psychosocial needs.

3. Demonstrate knowledge of legal and ethical obligations.

SIMULATION SCENARIO OBJECTIVES

1. Reflect on actions taken by self and peers, both civil and uncivil.

2. Apply the principles of trauma-informed care to individuals who identify as sexual minorities.

3. Discuss ways to create safe spaces and acceptance of LGBTQ individuals.

FOR FACULTY: REFERENCES, EVIDENCE-BASED PRACTICE GUIDELINES, PROTOCOLS, OR ALGORITHMS USED FOR THIS SCENARIO:

Meyer, I. H. (2003). Prejudice, social stress, and mental health in lesbian, gay, and bisexual populations: Conceptual issues and research evidence. *Psychological Bulletin, 129*(5), 674–697. doi: 10.1037/0033-2909.129.5.674

National LGBTQ Health Education Center (a program of the Fenway Institute). (n.d.). *LGBTQ health readiness assessments in health centers: Key findings*. Retrieved from https://www.lgbthealtheducation.org/wp-content/uploads/2017/11/LGBT-Health-Readiness-Assessment-Key-Findings.pdf

SETTING/ENVIRONMENT

Khris is changing into scrubs in the operating room (OR) staff area. Two other members of her clinical group are with her. They both observe that Khris has male anatomy, and one peer, Meredith, begins to giggle and whisper to the other student nurse, Laura. Khris is terrified of what will happen to her in school. The three students observe surgical cases and then arrive at post-conference with their clinical instructor, Dr. Thomas.

❏ Emergency Department	❏ ICU
❏ Medical-Surgical Unit	❏ OR/PACU
❏ Pediatric Unit	❏ Rehabilitation Unit
❏ Maternity Unit	❏ Home
❏ Behavioral Health Unit	❏ Outpatient Clinic
	☒ Other: Changing area in the OR; moves to post-clinical conference

EQUIPMENT/SUPPLIES

Simulated Patient/Manikins Needed: Standardized patients (2)

ROLES

GUIDELINES/INFORMATION RELATED TO ROLES

These roles will be filled by both standardized patients and student nurses participating in the simulation. The primary setting for this is the post-clinical conference room where each student nurse is reporting and being debriefed from their clinical experiences that morning.

- Khris: Standardized patient; student nurse whose male anatomy was observed when she was changing into scrubs for an observation experience in the OR

- Dr. Thomas: Standardized patient; clinical instructor

- Meredith: Standardized patient; student nurse and Khris's peer; behaves with incivility and ignorance

- Laura: Student nurse and Khris's peer; role may be taken by student

- Peers: Student peers, an additional three students who will primarily observe the interactions; roles may be taken by students

Khris's sexual identity will be exposed in front of the entire group prior to Dr. Thomas being able to stop Meredith, who describes her suspicions of Khris being a transgender young adult. Khris shuts down in front of the group. Dr. Thomas intervenes and uses trauma-informed communication to protect Khris from further traumatic stress. Laura also comes to Khris's defense and speaks to her talents as a nurse. At the end, Khris speaks to her peers about her past, which includes being a survivor of extreme bullying.

PREBRIEFING/BRIEFING (SEE STUDENT WORKBOOK)

While changing for a clinical observation day in the OR, one student nurse, Khris, is exposed as an MTF transgender individual. Meredith, one of the two peers who are in the changing room with Khris, discloses this to her entire clinical group. The clinical group is assembled with Dr. Thomas, their instructor, for their routine post-clinical conference. Dr. Thomas is unaware of the event in the OR changing room but notices that Meredith is whispering and giggling with other students. Khris is quiet and has isolated herself at the outer perimeter of the group. Dr. Thomas begins by asking the three students who observed in the OR, Khris, Meredith, and Laura, what they "saw in clinical today." Meredith bursts into a giggle.

The objectives of this simulation are to learn about civility and how to mitigate sexual minority stress through trauma-informed communications and actions.

REPORT STUDENTS WILL RECEIVE BEFORE SIMULATION

None

SCENARIO PROGRESSION OUTLINE

TIMING (APPROX.)	SP ACTIONS	EXPECTED INTERVENTIONS	MAY USE THE FOLLOWING CUES
0–5 mins	Meredith (SP) to Dr. Thomas (SP Instructor) "We saw a lot this morning!" Grins widely. Dr. Thomas: "It appears something is going on that I am unaware of. Meredith, please share with the rest of the group."	Learners should begin by: Watching group dynamics of clinical group. Observing verbal and nonverbal communications and interpreting meanings (support, incivility, power, and so on).	
5–10 mins	Meredith: "I'm not sure really. Ask Khris or Laura." Continues to grin, but looks down. Dr. Thomas turns to Khris and Laura: "Well??" Khris blurts out: "Everyone may as well know, since Meredith will make sure they do as soon as we leave this room: I'm a transgender individual. I was born biologically a male." Khris averts her eyes. "They saw me changing and noticed that I still retain some of the biological appearances of a male." Dr. Thomas: "I see. I also see..." she turns to Meredith, "that we haven't been very kind to you, Khris. I'm sorry for that. How did your peers' behavior affect you?" Khris remains silent.	Laura looks at Khris and moves to sit next to her.	
10–15 mins	Laura: "I think Khris's privacy and rights have been violated." She turns to Meredith: "You've been cruel, and I'm not sure why. You've disclosed something very personal—something that didn't belong to you to disclose." Laura continues: "I took care of a person who was transgender, and he had been through so much. He hadn't received the right care because we—members of the healthcare team—were uninformed and made assumptions we shouldn't have." Meredith stops grinning and crosses her arms.		Cue: Dr. Thomas encourages the others in the group to speak. Students should bring in information about sexual minorities and sexual minority stress.

TIMING (APPROX.)	SP ACTIONS	EXPECTED INTERVENTIONS	MAY USE THE FOLLOWING CUES
15–20 mins	Dr. Thomas, turning to Khris: "I want you to feel safe. It appears your peers support you. I support you. I hope you can learn to trust that safety."	Expect periods of silence.	
	Khris finally speaks again: "It's been hard. I suppose today was for the best. I've lived in a shadow world for a long time because so many in my family didn't understand me." She shakes her head and looks at Dr. Thomas: "I don't know how I feel."		
	Meredith, who now is sitting alone, says in a soft voice: "I'm sorry, Khris. I laugh when I'm uncomfortable. It's no excuse. But I didn't understand. I'm from a very conservative family."		
	General discussion ensues regarding family of orientation influences, clinical experiences, and implicit biases.		

DEBRIEFING/GUIDED REFLECTION

THEMES FOR THIS SCENARIO: SEXUAL MINORITY TRAUMA

Learner actions and responses observed by the debriefer should be specifically addressed using a theory-based debriefing methodology (such as Debriefing with Good Judgment, Debriefing for Meaningful Learning, or PEARLS). With a focus on Khris:

1. How did you feel throughout the simulation experience?

2. Give a brief summary of what happened in the simulation.

3. What were the main problems that you identified?

4. Discuss the knowledge and emotions guiding your thinking surrounding these main problems.

5. Discuss the information resources you used to support Khris. How did this guide your contributions in "post-conference"?

6. How did you and others communicate with Khris?

7. What specific issues would you want to take into consideration to provide for this peer's unique care needs?

8. Discuss the psychological safety issues you considered when engaging with Khris.

9. How would you assess the quality of trauma-informed care provided?

10. What could you do to improve the quality of this care?

---

11. If you were able to do this again, how would you handle the situation differently?

12. What did you learn from this experience?

13. How will you apply what you learned today to your clinical practice?

14. Is there anything else you would like to discuss?

Simulation Design Template (revised March 2018) © 2018, National League for Nursing. Originally adapted from Childs, Sepples, & Chambers (2007), Designing simulations for nursing education. In P. R. Jeffries (Ed.), *Simulation in nursing education: From conceptualization to evaluation* (pp. 42–58). Washington, DC: National League for Nursing.

Link to original template: https://sirc.nln.org/pluginfile.php/18733/mod_page/content/51/Simulation%20Design%20Template%20 2018.docx

POSTTRAUMATIC STRESS DISORDER: MILITARY VETERAN AND STUDENT

MARK SIMULATION

Mark is a 26-year-old army veteran who is enrolled in a two-year community college nursing program. After serving two deployments to Afghanistan where he saw active combat, he returned home one year ago. Due to a diagnosis of posttraumatic stress disorder (PTSD), Mark is in therapy to decrease his symptoms (recurrent nightmares and anxiety) and strengthen his marriage. After speaking with several career counselors, he decided to enroll in nursing school. Mark does not feel part of his student nursing community and is unsure whether entering school was the right decision. He is struggling, feeling he is conspicuous and isolated with little in common with his peers.

While in Afghanistan, Mark was part of five engagements with hostile forces. He saw several fellow soldiers injured in the fighting. He is in his freshman year and entering into a simulation lab for medical-surgical nursing. Today, the high-fidelity patient is to experience asystole, with a "code blue" called for resuscitation. The manikin and equipment are programmed to simulate the sights and sounds of a real code.

The focus of this simulation is not the code blue; rather, it is Mark, who experiences posttraumatic stress symptoms (PTSS) upon hearing the sounds of the monitor and code. His reaction is to shut down, situate his body against the wall, and become hypervigilant of any threats in the environment. For a time, he is unable to speak. As he begins to become more aware that there is no threat, he is embarrassed and has only a partial recollection of what has occurred.

SIMULATION 2

DISCIPLINE: Nursing

EXPECTED SIMULATION RUN TIME:
20–25 minutes

LOCATION: Simulation lab

TODAY'S DATE: _____

FILE NAME: Mark

STUDENT LEVEL: Undergraduate nursing student (freshman)

GUIDED REFLECTION TIME: Twice the amount of time that the simulation runs

LOCATION FOR REFLECTION: Simulation lab quiet room

BRIEF DESCRIPTION OF INDIVIDUAL

NAME: Mark Bandura

DATE OF BIRTH: 12/01/1992

GENDER: Male   **AGE:** 26 years   **WEIGHT:** 200 pounds   **HEIGHT:** 6'1"

RACE: White   **RELIGION:** Methodist

MAJOR SUPPORT: Wife; fellow veterans

PAST MEDICAL HISTORY: Freshman; fought in active combat and eliminated the enemy in several instances. Returned home approximately one year ago.

HISTORY OF PRESENT ILLNESS: In therapy x 6 months for PTSD

SOCIAL HISTORY: Mark is second-generation college; father and mother both retired military officers.

PRIMARY MEDICAL DIAGNOSIS: PTSD

SURGERIES/PROCEDURES & DATES: N/A

PSYCHOMOTOR SKILLS REQUIRED OF PARTICIPANTS PRIOR TO SIMULATION

None

COGNITIVE ACTIVITIES REQUIRED OF PARTICIPANTS PRIOR TO SIMULATION

PRIOR TO THE SIMULATION, THE STUDENT SHOULD:

WATCH THE VIDEO:

- Burke Jr., T. (2015). PTSD and returning to the classroom. TEDxYale. Retrieved from https://www.youtube.com/watch?v=XBGNJQWSYHY

READ:

Barry, A. E., Whiteman, S. D., & MacDermid Wadsworth, S. M. (2012). Implications of posttraumatic stress among military-affiliated and civilian students. *Journal of American College Health*, *60*(8), 562–573. doi: 10.1080/07448481.2012.721427

SIMULATION LEARNING OBJECTIVES

1. Employ strategies to reduce risk of harm to the peer.
2. Conduct assessments appropriate for the care of the peer in an organized and systematic manner.
3. Communicate with the peer in a manner that illustrates caring, reflects cultural awareness, and addresses psychosocial needs.
4. Make clinical judgments and decisions that are evidence-based.
5. Demonstrate knowledge of legal and ethical obligations.

SIMULATION SCENARIO OBJECTIVES

1. Assess for signs of PTSD within the context of veteran status.
2. Integrate knowledge of PTSD symptoms with trauma-informed assessment and immediate support.
3. Provide physical and psychological safety for the individual who is affected by a trauma trigger.

FOR FACULTY: REFERENCES, EVIDENCE-BASED PRACTICE GUIDELINES, PROTOCOLS, OR ALGORITHMS USED FOR THIS SCENARIO:

Review and select additional readings and videos (as appropriate):

- López, O. S., Springer, S. B., & Nelson, J. B. (2016). Veterans in the college classroom: Guidelines for instructional practices. *Adult Learning, 27*(4), 143–151. doi: 10.1177/1045159515601825

_____

- Military Family Research Institute at Purdue University. (n.d.). Our mission. Retrieved from https://www.mfri.purdue.edu/about-mfri-history/mission/
- National Center for PTSD: Department of Veterans Affairs. (2018). PTSDPubs: Search the article database. Retrieved from https://www.ptsd.va.gov/ptsdpubs/search_ptsdpubs.asp

SETTING/ENVIRONMENT

❏ Emergency Department	❏ ICU
❏ Medical-Surgical Unit	❏ OR/PACU
❏ Pediatric Unit	❏ Rehabilitation Unit
❏ Maternity Unit	❏ Home
❏ Behavioral Health Unit	❏ Outpatient Clinic
	☒ Other: Simulation Lab

EQUIPMENT/SUPPLIES

Simulated Patient/Manikins Needed: Manikin laying on bed; standardized patients (2)

Other Props & Moulage: The lab should be set up to simulate a code blue, which will be initiated for asystole. The lesson is to test the student nurses' knowledge in a code situation; however, the purpose of this simulation is to have the students recognize and appropriately intervene when a peer experiences a trauma trigger that results in PTSS.

Equipment Attached to Manikin/Simulated Patient:

- ☒ ID band
- ☒ IV tubing with primary line fluids running at __mL/hr
- ❏ Secondary IV line running at ___mL/hr
- ❏ IVPB with _____ running at mL/hr
- ❏ IV pump
- ❏ PCA pump
- ❏ Foley catheter with ___mL output
- ❏ 02
- ☒ Monitor attached
- ❏ Other:

Other Essential Equipment:

Medications and Fluids:

- ❏ Oral meds:
- ❏ IV fluids:
- ❏ IVPB:
- ☒ IV push:
- ❏ IM or SC:

Equipment Available in Room:

❑ Bedpan/urinal

❑ O2 delivery device (type)

❑ Foley kit

❑ Straight catheter kit

❑ Incentive spirometer

❑ Fluids

❑ IV start kit

❑ IV tubing

❑ IVPB tubing

❑ IV pump

❑ Feeding pump

☒ Crash cart with airway devices and emergency medications

☒ Defibrillator/pacer

❑ Suction

☒ Other: The sim room should be set up for a code blue; however, navigating a code is not the purpose of this simulation.

ROLES

☒ Student nurse 1: Mark, standardized patient

☒ Student nurse 2: Kayleigh, standardized patient

☒ Student nurse 3: Nicole

☒ Student nurse 4: Curt

☒ Provider (physician): Instructor who will initiate and terminate the code from the control room

❑ Other healthcare professionals: (pharmacist, respiratory therapist, and so on)

❑ Observer(s)

❑ Recorder(s)

❑ Family member #1

❑ Family member #2

❑ Clergy

❑ Unlicensed assistive personnel

❑ Other:

GUIDELINES/INFORMATION RELATED TO ROLES

Although the lab is equipped to simulate a code for a patient experiencing asystole, the monitor sounds and the students circling the bed and administering CPR will trigger posttraumatic stress symptoms of hypervigilance and anxiety in Mark, the standardized patient. Therefore, the primary setting is the simulation room with a focus on Mark's reactions:

- Mark: Standardized patient; student nurse who reacts to auditory and visual triggers in the environment (monitor and students' frantic efforts as asystole occurs)

- Dr. Adams: Clinical instructor who is running sim and instructing students; observes students through one-way mirror

- Kayleigh: Standardized patient; student nurse who observes Mark's distress and intervenes. She and Mark have become student buddies, and she is aware of his past military service.

- Nicole: Peer in clinical simulation; role may be taken by student

- Curt: Peer in clinical simulation; role may be taken by student

Mark's affect and physical appearance will change abruptly once the code is underway. The monitor and bodies circling the manikin will trigger PTSS in Mark. He will back into a wall, become unresponsive verbally, and be hypervigilant of his environment. Dr. Adams will emerge from the control room once these symptoms overwhelm the code and the students stop the simulation due to Mark's distress.

Students (peers) may assume the roles of clinical group members taking part in the simulation. They will be observed for how well and how quickly they notice Mark's withdrawal from the code activities, engage in assessing his condition, and take on trauma-informed interventions/communication.

PREBRIEFING/BRIEFING (SEE STUDENT WORKBOOK)

This simulation focuses on the team working during a code blue. One of the students' peers may not be able to continue with the simulation, and it is acceptable to end the code to render care to your peer.

The objective of this simulation is to become aware of how triggers of past traumatic events may affect individuals and how to respond in a therapeutic manner.

REPORT STUDENTS WILL RECEIVE BEFORE SIMULATION

Students will be advised that a code will be called for a heart anomaly. They will be required to be CPR certified and review basic code procedures.

SCENARIO PROGRESSION OUTLINE

TIMING (APPROX.)	SP ACTIONS	EXPECTED INTERVENTIONS	MAY USE THE FOLLOWING CUES
0–5 mins	Students circle the patient bed with a high-fidelity manikin. The manikin has a cardiac monitor in place with sounds audible from this monitor. One student initiates CPR with chest compressions. Another student begins to use an ambu bag with proper head placement for successful ventilations. A third student runs to bring the emergency cart to the bedside.	Learners should begin by: Noticing the cardiac arrhythmia and initiating CPR after asystole is called Observing Mark disengaging from group	Role member providing cue: Cue: Instructor from control room: "Patient is in asystole. Initiate CPR."
5–10 mins	Mark leaves the circle of the group and backs into a wall. CPR continues. Mark doesn't respond to the instructor's question.	Waiting to see how long it takes for a peer to notice Mark's distress	Cue: Instructor from control room: "Mark, are you OK?"
10–15 mins	Kayleigh: "Mark, are you OK?" Mark scans the room, brings arms up. He begins to breathe rapidly and perspire. Kayleigh: "Mark, it's me, Kayleigh. I'm in your clinical group. We're in the middle of a simulation. We're safe. This isn't real. There is nothing here to harm us."	Watching Kayleigh's and Mark's nonverbal behaviors Acknowledging that Kayleigh provides assurances for safety	Cue: Instructor from control room: "OK, guys, terminate the simulation."
15–20 mins	The other students come to Mark's side, but Kayleigh instructs them to be sure to "give him some space." She also assures the group that "things are OK." Kayleigh to Mark: "Let's sit down, OK?" She brings a chair for Mark and sits next to him. She waits for Mark's anxiety to lessen. After about three minutes, Mark looks around. "Wow. What just happened?" Kayleigh: "Well, I'm not sure, but something we did in the simulation may have reminded you of something in your past that was threatening or scary." Mark continues to appear to awaken from a trance. "Yeah." He becomes quiet and appears embarrassed.		Cue: Instructor emerges from the control room and waits for Kayleigh to indicate she needs help or for Mark to regain a sense of the here and now.

continues

SCENARIO PROGRESSION OUTLINE (CONT.)

TIMING (APPROX.)	SP ACTIONS	EXPECTED INTERVENTIONS	MAY USE THE FOLLOWING CUES
20–25 mins	Dr. Adams: "Let's move to the debriefing room and talk about this. Is that OK with you, Mark?" Mark nods. Dr. Adams begins to discuss what trauma triggers are. She is careful not to invade Mark's privacy; she wants to minimize Mark's feelings of embarrassment. Mark is encouraged to share: "I'll be honest. It's been tough. I feel different, you know. I guess today doesn't help." He grins in a sad way. Techniques such as summarizing, exploring, reflecting, restating, and other therapeutic techniques should be used as the student group and instructor continue to discuss the event and how each interpreted and reacted.	Students join Dr. Adams in the debriefing room, but the simulation is still occurring. The students need to observe how support is offered and provide it as appropriate.	Cue: Students process what the posttraumatic stress symptoms were and how students should use therapeutic communication techniques within a trauma-informed framework (provider and patient safety, trust, peer support, and so on).

DEBRIEFING/GUIDED REFLECTION

THEMES FOR THIS SCENARIO: PTSS: TRAUMA TRIGGERS

Learner actions and responses that the debriefer observes should be specifically addressed using a theory-based debriefing methodology (such as Debriefing with Good Judgment, Debriefing for Meaningful Learning, or PEARLS). With a focus on Mark:

1. How did you feel throughout the simulation experience?

2. Give a brief summary of this student nurse (Mark) and what happened in the simulation.

3. What were the key assessment and interventions for this peer?

4. Discuss how key assessments and interventions were identified.

5. How did you communicate with the individual in distress?

6. What specific issues would you want to take into consideration to provide for this individual's unique care needs?

7. Discuss the safety issues you considered when implementing care for this individual.

8. What measures did you implement to ensure safe care?

9. If you were able to do this again, how would you handle the situation differently?

10. What did you learn from this experience?

11. How will you apply what you learned today to your clinical practice?

12. Is there anything else you would like to discuss?

Simulation Design Template (revised March 2018) © 2018, National League for Nursing. Originally adapted from Childs, Sepples, & Chambers (2007), Designing simulations for nursing education. In P. R. Jeffries (Ed.), *Simulation in nursing education: From conceptualization to evaluation* (pp. 42–58). Washington, DC: National League for Nursing.

Link to original template: https://sirc.nln.org/pluginfile.php/18733/mod_page/content/51/Simulation%20Design%20Template%20 2018.docx

SECTION 2

TRAUMA DURING COLLEGE:
THE STUDENT NURSE AS CAREGIVER

SECOND-VICTIM TRAUMA: OVERWHELMED IN MED-SURG

Melanie is a junior in her baccalaureate nursing program and is in the first week of clinical. She needs to prepare and administer medications at 0900. Her first patient is a 67-year-old male with a history of alcohol dependency and atrial fibrillation. He was admitted for an emergency repair of an open femur fracture (open reduction internal fixation of the right distal femur) following a motor vehicular accident. Twelve hours post-operatively, the patient experienced an upper gastrointestinal bleed with hematemesis, confirmed with endoscopic examination, which revealed erosive disease. Melanie has made a serious medication error by administering warfarin to the patient.

In this simulation, the focus is Melanie, not Mr. Kline (the patient). The learning experience emphasizes second-victim trauma, which occurs after an adverse event that is typically attributed to provider error. Although apologies to the patient after such errors are recommended, the simulation time limits additional attention given to this. Students will be drawn to the empirical side of the error; however, Melanie's second-victim trauma should be the basis of the simulation.

SIMULATION 3

DISCIPLINE: Nursing

EXPECTED SIMULATION RUN TIME:
20–25 minutes

LOCATION: Simulation lab

TODAY'S DATE: _____

FILE NAME: Melanie

STUDENT LEVEL: Undergraduate nursing student (junior)

GUIDED REFLECTION TIME: Twice the amount of time that the simulation runs

LOCATION FOR REFLECTION: Simulation lab quiet room

BRIEF DESCRIPTION OF INDIVIDUAL

NAME: Joseph Kline

DATE OF BIRTH: 12/10/1951

GENDER: Male   **AGE:** 67 years   **WEIGHT:** 155 pounds   **HEIGHT:** 5'8"

RACE: White   **RELIGION:** Lutheran

MAJOR SUPPORT: AA sponsor   **SUPPORT PHONE:** AA sponsor

PAST MEDICAL HISTORY: Alcohol dependence (intermittent x 30 years), chronic atrial fibrillation, and hyperlipidemia

HISTORY OF PRESENT ILLNESS: Admitted through the ED post MVA during which patient suffered crushing injury to R distal femur and soft tissue injuries.

SOCIAL HISTORY: Patient is currently homeless.

PRIMARY MEDICAL DIAGNOSIS: Open fx R distal femur post MVA; post-surgical open reduction/internal fixation of R distal femur

SURGERIES/PROCEDURES & DATES: Open reduction/internal fixation R distal femur (October 29)

PSYCHOMOTOR SKILLS REQUIRED OF PARTICIPANTS PRIOR TO SIMULATION

None

COGNITIVE ACTIVITIES REQUIRED OF PARTICIPANTS PRIOR TO SIMULATION

PRIOR TO THE SIMULATION, THE STUDENT SHOULD:

WATCH THE VIDEO:

- Johns Hopkins Medicine. (2015). *The RISE program: Peer support for caregivers in distress.* Retrieved from https://www.youtube.com/watch?v=NiLEWpjNP6I

READ:

Delacroix, R. (2017). Exploring the experience of nurse practitioners who have committed medical errors: A phenomenological approach. *Journal of the American Association of Nurse Practitioners, 29*, 403–409. doi: 10.1002/2327-6924.12468

Scott, S. D., Hirschinger, L. E., Cox, K. R., McCoig, M., Hahn-Cover, K., Epperly, K. M., . . . Hall, L. W. (2010). Caring for our own: Deploying a systemwide second victim rapid response team. *The Joint Commission Journal on Quality and Patient Safety, 36*(5), 233–240.

Wu, A. W. (2000). The second victim: The doctor who makes the mistake needs help too. *BMJ, 320*(7237), 726–727.

SIMULATION LEARNING OBJECTIVES

1. Employ strategies to reduce risk of harm to the patient.

2. Perform priority nursing actions based on assessment and clinical data.

3. Reassess/monitor patient status following nursing interventions.

4. Communicate appropriately with other healthcare team members in a timely, organized, patient-specific manner.

5. Make clinical judgments and decisions that are evidence-based.

6. Practice within nursing scope of practice.

7. Demonstrate knowledge of legal and ethical obligations.

SIMULATION SCENARIO OBJECTIVES

1. Reflect on actions taken by self and peers as a medically adverse event unfolds.

2. Demonstrate trauma-informed communication techniques to support the provider who has made the error.

3. Deconstruct the error from an individual and systems approach with recommendations to prevent similar errors from occurring in the future.

FOR FACULTY: REFERENCES, EVIDENCE-BASED PRACTICE GUIDELINES, PROTOCOLS, OR ALGORITHMS USED FOR THIS SCENARIO:

Review and select additional readings and videos (as appropriate):

- Medically Induced Trauma Support Services. (2010). *Clinician support tool kit for healthcare.* Retrieved from http://mitss.org/wp-content/uploads/2017/11/Clinician-Support-Tool-Kit-for-Healthcare_05-07-2012.pdf

- Reising, D. L., & Hensel, D. (2014). Chapter 3: Clinical simulations focused on patient safety. In P. R. Jeffries (Ed.), *Clinical simulations in nursing education: Advanced concepts, trends, and opportunities* (pp. 22–43). Philadelphia, PA: National League of Nursing.

- Substance Abuse and Mental Health Services Administration. (2014). Guiding principles of trauma-informed care. *SAMHSA News, 22*(2). Retrieved from https://www.samhsa.gov/samhsaNewsLetter/Volume_22_Number_2/trauma_tip/guiding_principles.html

SETTING/ENVIRONMENT

❑ Emergency Department	❑ ICU
☒ Medical-Surgical Unit	❑ OR/PACU
❑ Pediatric Unit	❑ Rehabilitation Unit
❑ Maternity Unit	❑ Home
❑ Behavioral Health Unit	❑ Outpatient Clinic
	❑ Other:

EQUIPMENT/SUPPLIES

Simulated Patient/Manikins Needed: Standardized patients (2)

ROLES
GUIDELINES/INFORMATION RELATED TO ROLES

Although this pertains to a patient scenario, the patient plays a secondary role in this simulation. Therefore, the primary setting for this is the nurses station or outside the patient room:

- Melanie: Standardized patient; student nurse who makes a serious medical error (administers warfarin, which was on hold by physician order)

- Ms. Hawkins: Standardized patient; clinical instructor

- Sally: Unit staff nurse; role may be taken by student

- Dr. Dobson: Physician of Mr. Kline, who received incorrect medication; role may be taken by student

- Peers: Student peers who will offer support to Melanie

There will be considerable distress and emotion as the error is uncovered. Melanie will work with the instructor, also a standardized patient (Ms. Hawkins), who will react to the error and assist in filing an incident report.

Students (peers) may take on the roles of the unit staff nurse, Sally, who will call the physician, Dr. Dobson, to report the error. Dr. Dobson and Sally will speak on the phone. This could be performed on a speaker phone in a conference room with Melanie in attendance.

PREBRIEFING/BRIEFING (SEE STUDENT WORKBOOK)

Melanie, a student nurse on a medical-surgical clinical rotation, has made a serious medication error. She administered warfarin to Mr. Kline, who is recovering post-operatively. With a history of atrial fibrillation and prior to hospitalization, Mr. Kline had been prescribed warfarin 5 mg, PO, once daily.

All home medications had been continued in the hospital following surgery, including warfarin. Melanie administered the medication, despite knowing that Mr. Kline had experienced an upper GI bleed over the night shift. After administration, laboratory values revealed PT 49.6, INR 4.68, Hgb 5.4.

The objective of this simulation is to learn about second-victim trauma, which is experienced after a medical error, and ways to provide support to those making the error within a trauma-informed framework.

REPORT STUDENTS WILL RECEIVE BEFORE SIMULATION

TIME: 1000

PERSON PROVIDING REPORT: Melanie

SITUATION: Patient has received a potentially life-threatening dose of an anti-coagulant (recent upper GI bleed).

BACKGROUND: Melanie administered a medication unsafely to the patient, creating a potential life-threatening situation.

ASSESSMENT: Patient appears in no distress; vital signs normal; post-operative incision appears clean and intact. No signs of upper GI bleeding.

RECOMMENDATIONS: STAT PT, INR, CBC drawn; close monitoring for evidence of GI bleed; incident report filing; contact attending physician

SCENARIO PROGRESSION OUTLINE

PATIENT NAME: Mr. Kline   **DATE OF BIRTH:** 12/10/1951

TIMING (APPROX.)	SP ACTIONS	EXPECTED INTERVENTIONS	MAY USE THE FOLLOWING CUES
0–5 mins	Melanie (SP) to Ms. Hawkins (SP Instructor): "I've made a huge mistake" (starts to cry). "I gave Mr. Kline a medication that I shouldn't have." Ms. Hawkins, taking a breath, "Tell me exactly what happened." Pulls Melanie away from patient room to conference room.	Learners should begin by: Watching dynamics between Melanie and Ms. Hawkins Grasping context of medication error	Role member providing cue:
5–10 mins	Melanie and Ms. Hawkins continue to discuss situation. Joined by staff nurse, Sally, who is assigned to Mr. Kline. She is informed of error. Sally is upset and frustrated because this will require time in preparing an incident report, calling the attending physician, and performing additional monitoring of patient.	Student joins as Sally.	Ms. Hawkins should find and report to Sally.
10–15 mins	Sally, Ms. Hawkins, and Melanie proceed to room where there is a speaker phone to report the incident and receive any additional orders. Dr. Dobson is annoyed and concerned with Mr. Kline's risk for hemorrhage. He asks for vital signs, wound condition, and any evidence of bleeding. Asks: "How did this happen?" Melanie is quiet during the phone call, with Sally talking the most.	Student joins as Dr. Dobson.	If needed, go to the conference room to call the physician on speaker phone.
15–20 mins	Incident report is completed by Sally and Melanie and overseen by Ms. Hawkins.		
20–25 mins	The clinical experience has ended for the day. Melanie has been closely monitoring Mr. Kline, who has not had any signs of bleeding. She is relieved to be done with clinical, saying, "Maybe nursing just isn't for me. What if he dies?" Group dialogue continues with post-conference discussion of med errors and second-victim trauma.	Students join Melanie to offer peer support in post-conference (post-clinical). Ms. Hawkins is present.	Students process error with Melanie, who is still emotional about the incident. Students should use therapeutic communication techniques within a trauma-informed framework (provider and patient safety, trust, peer support, and so on).

DEBRIEFING/GUIDED REFLECTION

THEMES FOR THIS SCENARIO: SECOND-VICTIM TRAUMA

Learner actions and responses observed by the debriefer should be specifically addressed using a theory-based debriefing methodology (such as Debriefing with Good Judgment, Debriefing for Meaningful Learning, or PEARLS). With a focus on Melanie:

1. How did you feel throughout the simulation experience?

2. Give a brief summary of this patient and what happened in the simulation.

3. How do you think Melanie will feel during her next clinical experience?

4. What were the main problems that you identified?

5. Discuss the knowledge guiding your thinking surrounding these main problems.

6. Discuss the trauma-informed guiding principles and peer support shown toward Melanie.

7. Explain the nursing management considerations for this situation. Discuss the knowledge guiding your thinking.

8. Discuss the safety issues you considered when implementing care for this patient and for Melanie.

9. What measures should have been implemented to ensure safe patient care?

10. What other members of the care team should you consider important to achieving good care outcomes?

11. How would you assess the quality of care provided?

12. What could you do to improve the quality of care for this patient?

13. What did you learn from this experience?

14. How will you apply what you learned today to your clinical practice?

15. Is there anything else you would like to discuss?

Simulation Design Template (revised March 2018) © 2018, National League for Nursing. Originally adapted from Childs, Sepples, & Chambers (2007), Designing simulations for nursing education. In P. R. Jeffries (Ed.), *Simulation in nursing education: From conceptualization to evaluation* (pp. 42–58). Washington, DC: National League for Nursing.

Link to original template: https://sirc.nln.org/pluginfile.php/18733/mod_page/content/51/Simulation%20Design%20Template%20 2018.docx

SECONDARY TRAUMA WITH POSTTRAUMATIC STRESS SYMPTOMS: UNEXPECTED PATIENT DEATH

SAMUEL SIMULATION

Samuel (Sam) is a junior nursing student preparing to graduate next year. He is in his obstetric (OB) clinical rotation and is assigned to the Wright family: mom, Tracy, and dad, Tom. Tracy is a 41-week laboring primigravida. Her difficult labor lasts 39 hours and involves considerable bleeding and a third-degree episiotomy after the baby has passed through the birth canal. After a healthy infant girl is born, Tracy begins to lose an estimated 900 mL more blood. She is transferred to the intensive care unit for blood transfusions and monitoring. Sam is unable to accompany Tracy and stays with the newborn. Unfortunately, Sam learns from his clinical instructor, Dr. Schaffer, that Tracy passed due to postpartum hemorrhage. At the end of Sam's clinical experience, Tom returns to the nursery and cradles his daughter, sobbing uncontrollably. Sam provides emotional comfort and compassionate care.

In the subsequent days, Sam is awoken from sleep with the sounds of Tracy's screams while in labor. He feels anxious as his mid-semester clinical evaluation approaches. He really doesn't know whether nursing is going to be a good fit for him professionally.

The focus of the simulation is on Samuel's secondary trauma, despite Tom, who needs significant psychological support following the death of his wife and an understanding of postpartum hemorrhage. Students will be drawn to the empirical side of the event; however, Sam's secondary traumatic stress is the basis of the simulation. This focus will be enhanced by students learning about the concept of resilience and how this can be a buffer to secondary traumatic stress.

SIMULATION 4

DISCIPLINE: Nursing

EXPECTED SIMULATION RUN TIME:
15–20 minutes

LOCATION: Simulation lab

TODAY'S DATE: _____

FILE NAME: Samuel

STUDENT LEVEL: Undergraduate nursing student (junior)

GUIDED REFLECTION TIME: Twice the amount of time that the simulation runs

LOCATION FOR REFLECTION: Simulation lab quiet room

BRIEF DESCRIPTION OF INDIVIDUAL

NAME: Samuel Garcia

DATE OF BIRTH: 03/22/2000

GENDER: Male   **AGE:** 20 years   **WEIGHT:** 170 pounds   **HEIGHT:** 6'0"

RACE: Hispanic   **RELIGION:** Roman Catholic

MAJOR SUPPORT: Family   **FAMILY:** Parents

SOCIAL HISTORY: Sam is a first-generation college student. His goal of becoming a nurse is one he has internalized and one that his family and extended family want for him.

PSYCHOMOTOR SKILLS REQUIRED OF PARTICIPANTS PRIOR TO SIMULATION

None

COGNITIVE ACTIVITIES REQUIRED OF PARTICIPANTS PRIOR TO SIMULATION

PRIOR TO THE SIMULATION, THE STUDENT SHOULD:

WATCH THE VIDEO:

- Bormann, J. (2018). *Mantram, Session 1: What Mantram is and how to choose one.* PsychArmor Institute. Retrieved from https://www.youtube.com/watch?v=tyFRGpLJ9-4&index=3&list=PL5uXbOV BSV4X6xpPz79et7GcjdoMtioYx

Note that there are four sessions in this series.

_____

READ:

Garcia-Dia, M. J., DiNapoli, J. M., Garcia-Ona, L., Jakubowski, R., & O'Flaherty, D. (2013). Concept analysis: Resilience. *Archives of Psychiatric Nursing, 27*, 264–270. doi: http://dx.doi.org/10.1016/j.apnu.2013.07.003

Michalec, B., Diefenbeck, C., & Mahoney, M. (2013). The calm before the storm? Burnout and compassion fatigue among undergraduate nursing students. *Nurse Education Today, 33*, 314–320. doi: http://dx.doi.org/10.1016/j.nedt.2013.01.026

Niitsu, K., Houfek, J. F., Barron, C. R., Stoltengerg, S. F., Kupzyk, K. A., & Rice, M. J. (2017). A concept analysis of resilience integrating genetics. *Issues in Mental Health Nursing, 38*(11), 896–906. doi: 10.1080/01612840.2017.1350225

Substance Abuse and Mental Health Services Administration. (2014). *SAMHSA's concept of trauma and guidance for a trauma-informed approach.* HHS Publication No. (SMA) 14–4884. Rockville, MD: Author.

PERFORM SELF-ASSESSMENT: SECONDARY TRAUMATIC STRESS SCALE

See Table 3.2 (pages 73–74) in *The Influence of Psychological Trauma in Nursing.*

Bride, B. E., Robinson, M. M., & Yegidis, B. (2004). Development and validation of the Secondary Traumatic Stress Scale. *Research on Social Work Practice, 14*(1), 27–35. doi: 10.1177/1049731503254106

SIMULATION LEARNING OBJECTIVES

1. Employ strategies to reduce the risk of harm to peers.

2. Communicate with peers and the clinical instructor in a manner that illustrates caring, reflects cultural awareness, and addresses psychosocial needs.

3. Demonstrate knowledge of legal and ethical obligations.

SIMULATION SCENARIO OBJECTIVES

1. Identify the psychological reactions to secondary trauma.

2. Apply the three E's of trauma as outlined by SAMHSA (2014)— Event, Experience, Effects—to Sam's experience.

3. List two ways to integrate self-care into professional nursing practice.

FOR FACULTY: REFERENCES, EVIDENCE-BASED PRACTICE GUIDELINES, PROTOCOLS, OR ALGORITHMS USED FOR THIS SCENARIO:

American Psychiatric Association. (2013). Posttraumatic stress disorder: Diagnostic criteria. In *Diagnostic and Statistical Manual of Mental Disorders* (5th ed., pp. 271–280). Arlington, VA: Author.

Heise, B. A., Wing, D. K., & Hullinger, A. H. (2018). My patient died: A national study of nursing students' perceptions after experiencing a patient death. *Nursing Education Perspectives, 39*(6), 355–359. doi: 10.1097/01.NEP.0000000000000335

Morrison, L. E., & Joy, J. P. (2016). Secondary traumatic stress in the emergency department. *Journal of Advanced Nursing, 72*(11), 2894–2906. doi: 10.1111/jan.13030

SETTING/ENVIRONMENT

Sam is scheduled for his one-on-one mid-semester clinical evaluation. The quality of his work has decreased since Tracy's death. He is fatigued and hasn't been able to perform to minimal competencies in his obstetric nursing clinical course, with incomplete and unacceptable written work. Dr. Schaffer and he begin to discuss his clinical evaluation.

❑ Emergency Department	❑ ICU
❑ Medical-Surgical Unit	❑ OR/PACU
❑ Pediatric Unit	❑ Rehabilitation Unit
❑ Maternity Unit	❑ Home
❑ Behavioral Health Unit	❑ Outpatient Clinic
	☒ Other: Dr. Schaffer's faculty office

EQUIPMENT/SUPPLIES

Simulated Patient/Manikins Needed: Standardized patients (2)

ROLES

GUIDELINES/INFORMATION RELATED TO ROLE

Dr. Schaffer's role will be filled by a standardized patient; a standardized patient will also enact Sam's role in the simulation. The primary setting for this is the mid-semester clinical evaluation between Sam and Dr. Schaffer.

- Sam: Standardized patient; student nurse who is experiencing symptoms of PTSD and is currently failing the clinical course
- Dr. Schaffer: Standardized patient; clinical instructor
- Student peers will observe the interactions.

Dr. Schaffer understands that Sam was involved in a sudden, traumatic death of a patient. Initially, however, she doesn't appreciate the extent of how the experience has affected Sam. Dr. Schaffer's initial goal is to communicate to Sam that he is failing. In contrast, Sam is experiencing significant ambiguity about continuing in school and hasn't disclosed this to his major support system, his family.

PREBRIEFING/BRIEFING (SEE STUDENT WORKBOOK)

Sam has experienced a traumatic event—the unexpected death of a new mother—which has left him with symptoms of PTSD. He is failing the clinical course in obstetrical nursing and is unsure about continuing in nursing. Dr. Schaffer, his clinical instructor, is unaware of the extent of Sam's trauma.

The objectives of this simulation are to recognize the symptoms of PTSD in oneself and peers after witnessing others' trauma and to identify ways to mitigate secondary traumatic stress.

REPORT STUDENTS WILL RECEIVE BEFORE SIMULATION

None

SCENARIO PROGRESSION OUTLINE

TIMING (APPROX.)	SP ACTIONS	EXPECTED INTERVENTIONS	MAY USE THE FOLLOWING CUES
0–5 mins	Dr. Schaffer: "Have a seat, Sam." She sits across from him at her desk. Several papers are laid in front of her. She is wearing a lab coat. Sam appears anxious, yet disconnected. He avoids eye contact. Dr. Schaffer: "Let's start by my asking you: How do you think you're performing in this clinical course?" Sam: "OK, I guess." He appears confused and fidgets with a pen. Dr. Schaffer proceeds to point out the areas that Sam is deficient in, including graded assignments, such as concept maps and plans of care. She explains that for the first few weeks, Sam's performance had been strong.	Learners should begin by: Watching the nonverbal dynamics between Dr. Schaffer and Sam Observing verbal and nonverbal communications and interpreting meanings (support, confusion, anger, and so on)	

continues

SCENARIO PROGRESSION OUTLINE   (CONT.)

TIMING (APPROX.)	SP ACTIONS	EXPECTED INTERVENTIONS	MAY USE THE FOLLOWING CUES
5–10 mins	Dr. Schaffer pauses and looks at Sam. "Sam, are you understanding what I'm showing you?" Sam again mumbles, "I guess." Dr. Schaffer leans forward and waits. Sam continues to fidget with a pen and looks away. Dr. Schaffer pushes the papers aside and tries to make eye contact with Sam. "Let's back up a bit. About four weeks ago, you were part of a very sad and very unexpected patient trauma—the young mother who passed." Sam nods and whispers, "Tracy, Tom's wife and that little baby's mom." Taking a breath, Dr. Schaffer responds: "We discussed this in post-conference, but I know that witnessing that kind of trauma is very difficult and can cause trauma in those who render care." Sam finally makes eye contact. "I'm not sure about this whole nurse stuff to be honest. With what you're telling me, that kind of clinches it."	Watch for Dr. Schaffer's change in tone.	
10–15 mins	Dr. Schaffer appears to understand the response to Sam's experience. She goes on to question him about some of the symptoms of posttraumatic stress. Sam verifies that he's not sleeping, feels on alert all the time, and can't seem to shut his mind off.	Expect periods of silence from Sam, but more non-verbal engagement.	
15–20 mins	Dr. Schaffer then goes on to educate Sam about secondary trauma that nurses often experience. She also talks about compassion fatigue that may result from constant/chronic secondary trauma. Sam: "So how do you get around it? I mean, if it's part of the job, I don't think I can do this. And I don't want to get like some of those nurses I've seen on the floor. They have no expressions or are outright angry most of the time. I don't want to be like that. And if it's affecting me this much, I'm just not going to be a very good provider."	Look for assessment of the three E's of trauma: Event, Experience, and Effects.	

TIMING (APPROX.)	SP ACTIONS	EXPECTED INTERVENTIONS	MAY USE THE FOLLOWING CUES
15–20 mins (continued)	Dr. Schaffer looks kindly at Sam: "I can't deny most of what you just said, except this: I think you'll be a very good nurse. You care, Sam. Tracy's death had such an impact on you because you felt the overwhelming sadness of her husband and knew the loss to the child. We just have to figure out how to build your reserves, your resilience."		
	Dr. Schaffer goes on to describe her own compassion fatigue she had experienced years ago—fatigue from witnessing many patients' traumatic events. She talks about taking time to meditate, walk daily, and shut off technology, even if it meant others had to wait.		
	Sam nods slowly. "Maybe. I'll talk it over with my parents. They really want me to become a nurse."		
	Dr. Schaffer affirms this decision and ends by asking Sam questions to verify his psychological safety and a plan to improve his performance in class. She emphasizes that she is available to Sam if he needs to talk and offers him the contact information of the academic advisor and campus mental health resources.		

DEBRIEFING/GUIDED REFLECTION

THEMES FOR THIS SCENARIO: SECONDARY TRAUMA/SECONDARY TRAUMATIC STRESS

Learner actions and responses observed by the debriefer should be specifically addressed using a theory-based debriefing methodology (such as Debriefing with Good Judgment, Debriefing for Meaningful Learning, or PEARLS). With a focus on Sam:

1. How did you feel throughout the simulation experience?

2. Give a brief summary of this student and what happened in the simulation.

3. What were the main problems that you identified?

4. Discuss the knowledge guiding your thinking surrounding these main problems.

5. What were the key assessments and interventions for this student nurse?

6. Discuss how you identified these key assessments and interventions.

7. Discuss the information resources you used to assess this individual. How did this guide your care planning?

37

8. What specific issues would you want to take into consideration to provide for this student's unique care needs?

9. Discuss the safety issues you considered when implementing care for this student.

10. How would you assess the quality of interaction between Dr. Schaffer and Sam?

11. What could have been done to improve the quality of the interaction?

12. What did you learn from this experience?

13. How will you apply what you learned today to your clinical practice?

14. Is there anything else you would like to discuss?

Simulation Design Template (revised March 2018) © 2018, National League for Nursing. Originally adapted from Childs, Sepples, & Chambers (2007), Designing simulations for nursing education. In P. R. Jeffries (Ed.), *Simulation in nursing education: From conceptualization to evaluation* (pp. 42–58). Washington, DC: National League for Nursing.

Link to original template: https://sirc.nln.org/pluginfile.php/18733/mod_page/content/51/Simulation%20Design%20Template%20 2018.docx

SECTION 3

TRAUMA AFTER GRADUATION: BUILDING A RESILIENT NURSING WORKFORCE

SYSTEM-INDUCED TRAUMA

Rebecca is a 62-year-old elementary schoolteacher who had been experiencing ventricular tachycardia with brief periods (seconds) of unease and dizziness. She was admitted for cardiac ablation and transferred to ICU at one day post-cardiac ablation for uncontrolled bleeding from the femoral artery post-surgical procedure. Her bleeding stabilized after a blood transfusion, and she is due to be discharged tomorrow. There is currently no bleeding from the femoral catheter incision site, and there are no signs of infection.

Rebecca is adamant about "never going through something like that again!" She is asking to be discharged "ASAP!" because the hospital is a "deathtrap" and, more than likely, she'll "get some superbug that eats through my flesh." She is refusing morning care and respiratory therapy. (She is in early-stage congestive heart failure with a BMI of 31.) She also refuses to walk in the hallway and demands to know, prior to taking any medication, what its purpose is and why the physician prescribed it for her. Her husband sits in the room, silent.

In this simulation, the focus is on the trauma Rebecca has experienced during the ablation procedure and post-operative hemorrhage. She had not been prepared or educated properly on what would happen in the operating room during the ablation. Although she was consented by the surgeon, she did not fully realize what complications could occur or how they would be treated and where.

The nurses are impatient because they have other patients who need their care. Rebecca is taking precious time away from others due to her irrational demands and fears. Finally, the nurse manager, Holly, is called to speak with Rebecca as her behavior continues to escalate. Rebecca's nurse, Mary, is a new graduate and asked Holly to speak with Rebecca.

Described under various terms—medical trauma, system-induced trauma, and, when applicable, retraumatization—this simulation is designed to increase awareness of the effects of healthcare delivery on individuals. "Do no (psychological) harm" may be difficult given certain phenomena in healthcare today: staffing issues, high use of technology, and rapid turnover of inpatients.

SIMULATION 5

DISCIPLINE: Nursing

EXPECTED SIMULATION RUN TIME:
15–20 minutes

LOCATION: Simulation lab

TODAY'S DATE: _____

FILE NAME: Rebecca

STUDENT LEVEL: Undergraduate

GUIDED REFLECTION TIME: Twice the amount of time that the simulation runs

LOCATION FOR REFLECTION: Simulation lab quiet room

BRIEF DESCRIPTION OF INDIVIDUAL

NAME: Rebecca Jameston

DATE OF BIRTH: 02/20/1956

GENDER: Female   **AGE:** 62 years   **WEIGHT:** 180 pounds   **HEIGHT:** 5'3"

RACE: White   **RELIGION:** Christian

MAJOR SUPPORT: Husband   **SUPPORT PHONE:**

ALLERGIES: Sulfa drugs   **IMMUNIZATIONS:** Pneumovax vaccine due

ATTENDING PROVIDER/TEAM: Dr. Rush, cardiac surgeon; Holly, nursing supervisor post-cardiac surgery floor; Mary, newly licensed nurse

PAST MEDICAL HISTORY: Patient has had a fairly unremarkable medical history with annual physicals and wellness checks (mammograms, etc.). She has been diagnosed with early stage congestive heart failure, obesity (BMI = 31), and ventricular tachycardia (medication failed to reduce arrhythmia).

HISTORY OF PRESENT ILLNESS: Patient is one day post-cardiac ablation; refusing to adhere to post-op instructions (mobility and hygiene); blood pressure is increasing (130/85 at 0700; 140/90 at 1000). Becoming more agitated and verbally abusive toward staff.

SOCIAL HISTORY: Married 35 years

PRIMARY MEDICAL DIAGNOSIS: Post-cardiac ablation for ventricular tachycardia

SURGERIES/PROCEDURES & DATES: Cardiac ablation w/femoral catheter insertion

PSYCHOMOTOR SKILLS REQUIRED OF PARTICIPANTS PRIOR TO SIMULATION

None

COGNITIVE ACTIVITIES REQUIRED OF PARTICIPANTS PRIOR TO SIMULATION

PRIOR TO THE SIMULATION, THE STUDENT SHOULD:

WATCH THE VIDEO:

- Johns Hopkins Medicine. (2014). *ICU diaries help prevent PTSD: JHM piloting the initiative.* Retrieved from https://www.youtube.com/watch?v=abMPULXpUVw

READ:

Marsac, M. L., Kassam-Adams, N., Delahanty, D. L., Widaman, K. F., & Barakat, L. P. (2014). Posttraumatic stress following medical trauma in children: A proposed model of bio-psycho-social processes during the peri-trauma period. *Clinical Child and Family Psychological Review, 17*, 399–411. doi: 10.1007/s10567-014-0174-2

Walz, G. R., & Bleuer, J. C. (2013). When treatment becomes trauma: Defining, preventing, and transforming medical trauma. *VISTAS Online,* Article 73. Retrieved from https://www.counseling.org/docs/default-source/vistas/when-treatment-becomes-trauma-defining-preventing-.pdf

SIMULATION LEARNING OBJECTIVES

1. Employ strategies to reduce the risk of further harm to the patient.

2. Conduct assessments appropriate for patient care in an organized and systematic manner.

3. Perform priority nursing actions based on assessment and clinical data.

4. Reassess/monitor the patient status following nursing interventions.

5. Communicate with the patient and the family in a manner that illustrates caring, reflects cultural awareness, and addresses psychosocial needs.

6. Communicate appropriately with other healthcare team members in a timely, organized, patient-specific manner.

7. Make clinical judgments and decisions that are evidence-based.

8. Practice within nursing scope of practice.

9. Demonstrate knowledge of legal and ethical obligations.

SIMULATION SCENARIO OBJECTIVES

1. Recognize the signs and symptoms of medical trauma experienced by those who have been treated in ICU, which could lead to unfair labeling of patient behaviors.

2. Design interventions that mitigate PTSS experienced by patients post-ICU.

3. Within a traumatic stress framework, use therapeutic communication techniques to raise patient awareness of their experiences.

FOR FACULTY: REFERENCES, EVIDENCE-BASED PRACTICE GUIDELINES, PROTOCOLS, OR ALGORITHMS USED FOR THIS SCENARIO:

Review and select additional readings:

Parker, A. M., Sricharoenchai, T., Raparla, S., Schneck, K. W., Bienvenu, O. J., & Needham, D. M. (2015). Posttraumatic stress disorder in critical illness survivors: A metaanalysis. *Critical Care Medicine, 43*(5), 1121–1129. doi: 10.1097/CCM.0000000000000882

Roberts, M. B., Glaspey, L. J., Mazzarelli, A., Jones, C. W., Kilgannon, H. J., Trzeciak, S., & Roberts, B. W. (2018). Early interventions for the prevention of posttraumatic stress symptoms in survivors of critical illness: A qualitative systematic review. *Critical Care Medicine, 46*(8), 1328–1333. doi: 10.1097/CCM.0000000000003222

SETTING/ENVIRONMENT

❑ Emergency Department	☒ ICU
❑ Medical-Surgical Unit	❑ OR/PACU
❑ Pediatric Unit	❑ Rehabilitation Unit
❑ Maternity Unit	❑ Home
❑ Behavioral Health Unit	❑ Outpatient Clinic
	❑ Other:

EQUIPMENT/SUPPLIES

Simulated Patient/Manikins Needed: Standardized patient (1)

Equipment Attached to Manikin/Simulated Patient:

☒ ID band

☒ IV tubing with primary line fluids running at __mL/hr

❑ Secondary IV line running at ___mL/hr

❑ IVPB with _____ running at mL/hr

❑ IV pump

❑ PCA pump

❑ Foley catheter with ___mL output

❑ O2

☒ Monitor attached

❑ Other:

Other Essential Equipment:

Medications and Fluids:

☒ Oral meds:

❑ IV fluids:

❑ IVPB:

❑ IV push:

❑ IM or SC:

Equipment Available in Room:

❑ Bedpan/urinal

❑ O2 delivery device (type)

❑ Foley kit

❑ Straight catheter kit

❑ Incentive spirometer

❑ Fluids

❑ IV start kit

❑ IV tubing

❑ IVPB tubing

❑ IV pump

❑ Feeding pump

❑ Crash cart with airway devices and emergency medications

❑ Defibrillator/pacer

❑ Suction

❑ Other: The sim room should be set up for a code blue; however, navigating a code is not the purpose of this simulation.

ROLES

☒ Nurse 1 Holly, nurse manager

☒ Nurse 2 Mary, staff nurse

❑ Nurse 3

❑ Provider (physician/advanced practice nurse)

☒ Other healthcare professionals: Respiratory therapist

❑ Observer(s)

❑ Recorder(s)

☒ Family member #1 Bill, patient's husband

❑ Family member #2

❑ Clergy

❑ Unlicensed assistive personnel

❑ Other

GUIDELINES/INFORMATION RELATED TO ROLES

The primary setting for this is the patient room in ICU.

- Rebecca: Standardized patient who is experiencing PTSS, which are translating into abusive behaviors toward the staff

- Holly: ICU nurse manager; role may be taken by student or advanced nursing student

- Mary: Staff nurse assigned to Rebecca; role may be taken by student

- Respiratory therapist: In room, trying to coax Rebecca into her therapy; role may be taken by student

- Bill, Rebecca's husband: In room, mostly silent; role may be taken by student

Rebecca is demonstrating considerable agitation and appears emotionally distraught. However, as Holly begins to use trauma-informed language and techniques, Rebecca calms down, and her husband, Bill, begins to speak.

Students may take on the roles of Holly, Mary, the respiratory therapist, and Bill.

PREBRIEFING/BRIEFING (SEE STUDENT WORKBOOK)

Rebecca was admitted for a cardiac ablation procedure to treat her ventricular tachycardia on Monday. She was due to be discharged on Tuesday; however, because of a femoral bleed, the insertion site of the catheter used in the procedure, she received 6 units of whole blood, and her hospital stay was extended by two days. She is due to be discharged tomorrow but first needs to walk down the hall with minimal assistance and participate in her care.

The objective of this simulation is to learn about system-induced or medical trauma. This type of trauma is experienced due to care rendered and as the aftereffects of such care are realized. Interpreting patient behaviors within this context is the focus of this activity.

REPORT STUDENTS WILL RECEIVE BEFORE SIMULATION

TIME: 1100; readying patient for discharge

PERSON PROVIDING REPORT: Mary, patient's staff nurse

SITUATION: Patient being discharged tomorrow. Needs to walk down hall and toilet with minimal assistance. Husband at bedside. Vitals: blood pressure increasing. Patient agitated and behavior is escalating.

BACKGROUND: Patient has been in ICU x 3 days post cardiac ablation and hemorrhage at femoral catheter insertion site. Received 6 units whole blood in ICU post ablation d/t hemorrhage at femoral catheter insertion site. Current labs: Hgb = 11.1

ASSESSMENT: Patient is stable overall. B/P is currently 140/90, increasing with patient agitation. Demanding immediate discharge. Considering AMA discharge.

RECOMMENDATION: Request unit manager speak with patient.

SCENARIO PROGRESSION OUTLINE

TIMING (APPROX.)	SP ACTIONS	EXPECTED INTERVENTIONS	MAY USE THE FOLLOWING CUES
0–5 mins	Holly enters Rebecca's ICU room, and Mary enters a short time later. Holly notes Bill, who is sitting quietly at the end of the room, leaning against the window. Holly extends her hand to both Rebecca and Bill, introducing herself. Holly: "How are you feeling, Rebecca?" Rebecca sits in a patient chair with a lap cover over her knees and a breakfast tray that is relatively untouched. Monitors are running, and an IV is hooked to her left arm. She appears disheveled. "Not good. I want out of here NOW!" Holly pulls an extra chair up to Rebecca's side and slowly sits down beside her. "I've reviewed some notes about your hospital stay. It looks as if you've really been through a lot. Much of what you've experienced was unexpected and unknown to you. But why don't you tell me what happened to you."	Learners should begin by: Watching the nonverbal dynamics of Holly, Mary, Rebecca, and Bill Observing verbal and nonverbal communications and interpreting meanings (support, confusion, anger, and so on)	Note: Holly is using SAMHSA's recommended language for trauma survivors: "What happened to you?" vs. "What is wrong with you?" Holly does NOT bring up problematic behaviors or why she has been asked to talk with her.
5–10 mins	Rebecca pauses because she did not expect someone to ask this question or acknowledge her traumatic experiences. Rebecca, still very angry: "It's been awful. And I'm so horrified by it all." Holly: "Help me understand." Rebecca: "I remember lying on the OR cart and vaguely hearing my doctor's voice and then, more urgent voices, talking about getting units of blood. Losing control of my body. Being treated like a body, with no voice or soul. I thought I was dying." She begins to sob. Rebecca murmurs: "No one told me about any of this... I just want to go home. If I'm going to die, that's where I want to be."	Watching for Rebecca to deescalate Recording the effect of the language on the individual who has experienced trauma	

continues

SCENARIO PROGRESSION OUTLINE   (CONT.)

TIMING (APPROX.)	SP ACTIONS	EXPECTED INTERVENTIONS	MAY USE THE FOLLOWING CUES
10–15 mins	Bill walks over to put his hand on Rebecca's shoulder. Holly: "There's lots of good news I need to try to convey to you." She looks at her notes. "Your labs are stable, and you seem to have good mobility. Overall, since the time you needed blood, your recovery has been smooth." Rebecca starts to respond angrily. "SO what you're saying…" Holly gently but firmly states: "What I'm saying is that we have the same goal: to have you return home to heal. And that I hope you can begin to feel safe. I know you lost that sense of safety earlier when things happened after surgery that were unexpected."	Expect Bill to become more engaged. Mary adjusts Rebecca's IV tubing and looks at the monitors.	
15–20 mins	Holly begins to include Bill: "You've been through a lot as well." Bill tears up. "We've been married a long time. I don't know what I'd do without her." Holly acknowledges this feeling: "It must have been so frightening for both of you." Holly continues this dialogue with Rebecca and Bill. She sends messages of hearing their voices and tries to build trust. She emphasizes mutual goals, but there are behaviors that Rebecca needs to demonstrate—related to her recovery and her emotional regulation—to meet these goals. At the end of the discussion, Rebecca is tired, but she is no longer agitated or demanding. She apologizes to Mary. Mary: "It's OK. I'm glad you're feeling better." Holly: "I'm going to leave now, but Mary can let me know if you'd like to talk more later. I leave at about 6 this evening, but I'm here all day. Your doctor should be in soon to see you as well." Bill thanks both nurses and is engaged with Rebecca.	Look for assessment of the three E's of trauma: Event, Experience, and Effects.	

DEBRIEFING/GUIDED REFLECTION

THEMES FOR THIS SCENARIO: SYSTEM-INDUCED OR MEDICAL TRAUMA

Learner actions and responses observed by the debriefer should be specifically addressed using a theory-based debriefing methodology (such as Debriefing with Good Judgment, Debriefing for Meaningful Learning, or PEARLS). With a focus on Rebecca:

1. How did you feel throughout the simulation experience?

2. Give a brief summary of this patient and what happened in the simulation.

3. What were the main problems that you identified?

4. Discuss the knowledge guiding your thinking surrounding these main problems.

5. What were the key assessment and interventions for this patient?

6. Discuss how you identified these key assessments and interventions.

7. Explain the nursing management considerations for this patient. Discuss the knowledge guiding your thinking.

8. What specific issues would you want to take into consideration to provide for this patient's unique care needs?

9. Discuss the safety issues you considered when implementing care for this patient.

10. What measures did you implement to ensure safe patient care?

11. What other members of the care team should you consider important to achieving good care outcomes?

12. How would you assess the quality of care provided?

13. If you were able to do this again, how would the nurses handle the situation differently?

14. What did you learn from this experience?

15. How will you apply what you learned today to your clinical practice?

16. Is there anything else you would like to discuss?

Simulation Design Template (revised March 2018) © 2018, National League for Nursing. Originally adapted from Childs, Sepples, & Chambers (2007), Designing simulations for nursing education. In P. R. Jeffries (Ed.), *Simulation in nursing education: From conceptualization to evaluation* (pp. 42–58). Washington, DC: National League for Nursing.

Link to original template: https://sirc.nln.org/pluginfile.php/18733/mod_page/content/51/Simulation%20Design%20Template%202018.docx

WORKPLACE VIOLENCE

An emergency department (ED) nurse, Lizzie, was seriously injured by a patient on ecstasy. As a result of the attack, Lizzie suffered a concussion, broken jaw, and two broken ribs. After eight weeks, she has been released to resume employment, but is struggling in her performance. Her co-workers have been complaining to the ED manager, Carol, that Lizzie has been "slacking" and unengaged with patients, forcing other nurses to cover for her, and frequently calling off.

This simulation pertains to the traumatic experience that Lizzie is processing. Her primary way of coping with her posttraumatic stress is to avoid situations that she feels unsafe in, creating more work for her peers and, at times, creating safety issues for patients left unattended. Carol decides to speak with Lizzie as a trauma-informed supervisor.

SIMULATION 6

DISCIPLINE: Nursing

EXPECTED SIMULATION RUN TIME:
15–20 minutes

LOCATION: Simulation area or classroom

TODAY'S DATE: _____

FILE NAME: Lizzie

STUDENT LEVEL: Undergraduate

GUIDED REFLECTION TIME: Twice the amount of time that the simulation runs

LOCATION FOR REFLECTION: Simulation lab quiet room

BRIEF DESCRIPTION OF INDIVIDUAL

NAME: Lizzie Turner

DATE OF BIRTH: 03/15/1996

GENDER: Female   **AGE:** 24 years   **WEIGHT:** 119 pounds   **HEIGHT:** 5'4"

RACE: White   **RELIGION:** Baptist

MAJOR SUPPORT: Parents and boyfriend   **SUPPORT PHONE:**

TEAM: Carol, ED nurse manager

PAST MEDICAL HISTORY: Healthy adult who has prided herself in being physically fit. Avid runner who has competed in marathons.

HISTORY OF PRESENT ILLNESS: Patient became increasingly agitated in ED and attacked Lizzie who suffered a concussion, broken lower mandible, and two cracked ribs. Recently has lost 10 pounds due to jaw being wired shut and pain from ribcage. Weaning off pain medications and discomfort is currently controlled with NSAIDs. Residual vertigo from concussion is diminishing.

SOCIAL HISTORY: In committed relationship with boyfriend of two years; parents reside in same city as Lizzie and are supportive.

PRIMARY MEDICAL DIAGNOSIS: Post-concussion, lower mandible fracture with jaw wiring and two right cracked ribs

SURGERIES/PROCEDURES & DATES: Oral surgery September 12 (one day post-assault); on paid leave from work eight weeks

PSYCHOMOTOR SKILLS REQUIRED OF PARTICIPANTS PRIOR TO SIMULATION

None

COGNITIVE ACTIVITIES REQUIRED OF PARTICIPANTS PRIOR TO SIMULATION

PRIOR TO THE SIMULATION, THE STUDENT SHOULD:

READ:

National Child Traumatic Stress Network. (2018). *Using the secondary traumatic stress core competencies in trauma-informed supervision.* Retrieved from https://www.nctsn.org/sites/default/files/resources/fact-sheet/using_the_secondary_traumatic_stress_core_competencies_in_trauma-informed_supervision.pdf

Speroni, K. G., Fitch, T., Dawson, E., Dugan, L., & Atherton, M. (2014). Incidence and cost of nurse workplace violence perpetrated by hospital patients or patient visitors. *Journal of Emergency Nursing, 40*(3), 218–228. doi: https://doi.org/10.1016/j.jen.2013.05.014

Wei, C-Y., Chiou, S-T., Chien, L-Y., & Huang, N. (2016). Workplace violence against nurses—Prevalence and association with hospital organizational characteristics and health-promotion efforts: Cross-sectional study. *International Journal of Nursing Studies, 56*, 63–70. doi: http://dx.doi.org/10.1016/j.ijnurstu.2015.12.012

Zhang, L., Wang, A., Xiec, X., Zhouc, Y., Lid, J., Yange, L., & Zhang, J. (2017). Workplace violence against nurses: A cross-sectional study. *International Journal of Nursing Studies, 72*, 8–14. doi: https://doi.org/10.1016/j.ijnurstu.2017.04.002

ENROLL IN COURSE ON WORKPLACE VIOLENCE:

National Institute for Occupational Safety and Health: Centers for Disease Control and Prevention. (2016). Workplace violence prevention for nurses. Retrieved from https://wwwn.cdc.gov/wpvhc/Course.aspx/Slide/Intro_2

SIMULATION LEARNING OBJECTIVES

1. Employ strategies to reduce risk of harm to the nurse.
2. Conduct assessments appropriate for nursing care in an organized and systematic manner.
3. Perform priority nursing actions based on assessment and clinical data.
4. Reassess/monitor nurse status following interventions.
5. Communicate with the nurse in a manner that illustrates caring, reflects cultural awareness, and addresses psychosocial needs.
6. Communicate appropriately with other healthcare team members in a timely, organized, patient-specific manner.
7. Make supervisory and clinical judgments and decisions that are evidence-based.
8. Demonstrate knowledge of legal and ethical obligations.

SIMULATION SCENARIO OBJECTIVES

1. Design a therapeutic discussion between a nurse who has experienced workplace violence and a trauma-informed supervisor.
2. Substitute nontherapeutic dialogue with appropriate dialogue when counseling a nurse who has experienced trauma related to workplace violence.
3. Build strategies to support personal safety when rendering care to patients and their families.

FOR FACULTY: REFERENCES, EVIDENCE-BASED PRACTICE GUIDELINES, PROTOCOLS, OR ALGORITHMS USED FOR THIS SCENARIO:

Review and select additional readings:

The Joint Commission. (April 18, 2018). The Joint Commission issues new sentinel event alert on violence against health care workers during Workplace Violence Awareness Month. Retrieved from https://www.jointcommission.org/the_joint_commission_issues_new_sentinel_event_alert_on_violence_against_health_care_workers_during_workplace_violence_awareness_month/

SETTING/ENVIRONMENT

❏ Emergency Department	❏ ICU
❏ Medical-Surgical Unit	❏ OR/PACU
❏ Pediatric Unit	❏ Rehabilitation Unit
❏ Maternity Unit	❏ Home
❏ Behavioral Health Unit	❏ Outpatient Clinic
	☒ Other: Nurse manager's office

EQUIPMENT/SUPPLIES

Simulated Patient/Manikins Needed: Standardized patient (1)

ROLES

☒ Nurse 1: Carol, nurse manager	❏ Recorder(s)
☒ Nurse 2: Lizzie, newly returned to work	❏ Family member #1
❏ Nurse 3	❏ Family member #2
❏ Provider (physician/advanced practice nurse)	❏ Clergy
❏ Other healthcare professionals: (pharmacist, respiratory therapist, and so on)	❏ Unlicensed assistive personnel
	❏ Other
❏ Observer(s)	

GUIDELINES/INFORMATION RELATED TO ROLES

The primary setting for this is the nurse manager's office embedded in the ED.

- Carol: Standardized patient and ED nurse manager

- Lizzie: ED nurse who is experiencing difficulties in returning to her professional role post workplace violence. A student nurse may take this role.

Lizzie has been demonstrating behaviors consistent with avoidance post trauma. If there is an option, she requests female patients and has been calling off multiple times over the past few weeks. Her peers have been complaining to Carol about Lizzie's lack of teamwork and report multiple occasions when they were not able to locate Lizzie. They also report what seems to be "mood swings" when they talk to Lizzie.

Lizzie is defensive initially. Students observe Carol's use of supervisor competencies when interacting with employees who have experienced trauma (note that the competencies in the readings are for secondary traumatic stress; in this simulation, there is direct trauma to the nurse).

PREBRIEFING/BRIEFING (SEE STUDENT WORKBOOK)

Lizzie was called into Carol's office for a discussion following her return from a workplace violence injury. Lizzie is considering leaving the organization and perhaps even leaving nursing. Her recovery from the injuries has been difficult and emotionally exhausting. She has intrusive thoughts about the patient lunging toward her; the second just prior to contact is frozen in her memory. She cannot forget the image of the patient's face as he reaches out for her. The actual event plays over and over in her mind, with recurrent thoughts of self-recrimination and how she should have been more alert given the report from the policemen who brought the patient to the ED.

Carol is aware of Lizzie's experiences and injuries and hopes to find ways to strengthen Lizzie's feelings of safety, emotional regulation, and social connections.

The objective of this simulation is to learn about the posttraumatic stress symptoms following workplace violence/injury. The simulation also brings forth an appreciation of a trauma-informed nursing supervisor and the support offered to employees who have experienced a traumatic event.

SCENARIO PROGRESSION OUTLINE

TIMING (APPROX.)	SP ACTIONS	EXPECTED INTERVENTIONS	MAY USE THE FOLLOWING CUES
0–5 mins	Lizzie knocks on Carol's door. She seems fidgety: "You had asked me to come by." Carol moves from behind the desk to sit next to Lizzie: "Yes, please come in." Lizzie avoids eye contact. Carol: "How are you doing today?" Lizzie: "OK." Carol: "I know these past few months haven't been easy for you…" Lizzie nods. There's silence for several seconds. Carol: "Can you tell me what happened to you— in a way that feels safe for you—and what has happened since returning to work?" Lizzie: "What do you mean, 'safe'?" Carol: "I mean you can summarize, or you can go over certain events in more detail. You decide what is comfortable for you. I want to understand what you've experienced without causing you more discomfort."	Learners should begin by: Watching nonverbal dynamics between Carol and Lizzie Note: Identify how Carol is using core competencies for supervisors.	
5–10 mins	Finally, Lizzie opens up about the patient attack. At times, she is very emotional (cries), and at times, she is solemn and flat. She describes how she had to undergo oral surgery and lost weight and couldn't work out, making her feel even more physically vulnerable. Lizzie ends by saying: "I know the others think I've grown lazy and I'm not helping out like I used to." Carol: "You've been through so much. And the ways to treat your injuries made you feel less safe." Lizzie: "Exactly! I know I'm not functioning as I should. Maybe I should resign."	Watch for Lizzie to have some emotional dysregulation. Look for assessment of the three E's of trauma: Event, Experience, and Effects.	

TIMING (APPROX.)	SP ACTIONS	EXPECTED INTERVENTIONS	MAY USE THE FOLLOWING CUES
10–15 mins	Carol: "Well, let's slow things down. The ED is a unique place to work, and it's becoming a place where the most vulnerable come for services. Unfortunately, some of them inflict harm on those who are trying to help them."	Expect Carol to offer choices and feedback to Lizzie.	
	Lizzie tears up.		
	Carol: "I want to share with you that I was also hurt by a patient about four years ago."		
	Lizzie: "Really? What happened?"		
	Carol relates how an older patient with dementia bit her on the arm, requiring stitches and antibiotics. "It was traumatic for me. It seemed like such an animalistic way to harm someone."		
	Lizzie: "How did you get over it?"		
	Carol: "I had a good supportive network, but it took some time. I shared freely how much it had impacted me. I saw a counselor for a while. I processed anger, fear, not feeling safe, feeling different, and even guilt. At times, my emotions were all over the place."		
15–20 mins	Carol and Lizzie continue to talk. In this discussion, Carol does the following:	Look for assessment of the three E's of trauma: Event, Experience, and Effects.	
	Explores the financial option of having Lizzie reduce her schedule by one shift per week to allow more time to heal.		
	Describes employee assistance to facilitate counseling either within the organization or through external resources.		
	Outlines what Lizzie feels comfortable disclosing to peers so that they understand her behaviors and seek ways to support her feelings of safety.		
	Instructs Lizzie to enroll in the National Institute for Occupational Safety and Health (NIOSH) free online course to empower her efforts to prevent future workplace violence and protect herself.		
	Informs Lizzie about resiliency and how it can be fostered, as well as posttraumatic growth.		

DEBRIEFING/GUIDED REFLECTION

THEMES FOR THIS SCENARIO: WORKPLACE VIOLENCE

Learner actions and responses observed by the debriefer should be specifically addressed using a theory-based debriefing methodology (such as Debriefing with Good Judgment, Debriefing for Meaningful Learning, or PEARLS). With a focus on Lizzie and Carol:

1. How did you feel throughout the simulation experience?

2. Give a brief summary of Lizzie's experiences and what happened in the simulation.

3. What were the main problems that you identified?

4. Discuss the knowledge guiding your thinking surrounding these main problems.

5. What were the key assessment and interventions for Lizzie's performance and personal trauma?

6. Discuss how you identified these key assessments and interventions.

7. Discuss the information resources you used to assess Lizzie's situation. How did this guide your care planning?

8. Explain the nursing management considerations in this situation. Discuss the knowledge guiding your thinking.

9. How did Carol communicate with Lizzie? Do you agree with her choice to share her own trauma history?

10. What specific issues would you want to take into consideration to provide for Lizzie's unique needs?

11. What other members of the care team should you consider important to achieving good outcomes for Lizzie?

12. How would you assess the quality of the interaction?

13. What could you do to improve the quality of the discussion?

14. What did you learn from this experience?

15. How will you apply what you learned today to your clinical practice?

16. Is there anything else you would like to discuss?

Simulation Design Template (revised March 2018) © 2018, National League for Nursing. Originally adapted from Childs, Sepples, & Chambers (2007), Designing simulations for nursing education. In P. R. Jeffries (Ed.), *Simulation in nursing education: From conceptualization to evaluation* (pp. 42–58). Washington, DC: National League for Nursing.

Link to original template: https://sirc.nln.org/pluginfile.php/18733/mod_page/content/51/Simulation%20Design%20Template%20 2018.docx

ENDING THOUGHTS ON PEDAGOGY AND TRAUMA SIMULATIONS

By now, we hope you've noticed a theme in the simulations we've presented. The theme is this: The nurse, as a person and professional, needs care post trauma. As we pour ourselves, our knowledge, and our therapeutic use of self into our care, we often don't extend this care to self and peers. We don't see ourselves as recipients of compassion, and this needs to change. We can provide significant support for one another at the right time in the right place. We need to extend our talents to one another, especially with our professional world being so crowded with trauma. While these simulations don't depend on technology as many simulation activities do, we believe they offer faculty and students opportunities to learn and practice critical skills—and as importantly—prepare for situations that involve the different forms of trauma patients and peers are exposed to.

POSTTRAUMATIC GROWTH

One theme to be aware of as a facilitator in simulation learning is to expose your students to the idea of post-traumatic growth and building resiliency. Obviously, it is not a matter of *whether* students and new nurses will be confronted with trauma directly or as secondary trauma; it is a matter of when and how frequently. As such, you need to remind students that at the end of the process of recovery from trauma, individuals may grow internally, as well as have increased resiliency and inner strength. We believe this will translate to more compassionate, attuned care to vulnerable patients.

www.ingramcontent.com/pod-product-compliance
Lightning Source LLC
Chambersburg PA
CBHW080405270326
41927CB00015B/3353